Haematology
Lecture Notes

Chris S.R. Hatton

FRCP, FRCPath
Consultant Haematologist
Department of Haematology
The John Radcliffe Hospital, Oxford

Nevin C. Hughes-Jones

DM, PhD, MA, FRCP, FRS
Former Member of the Scientific Staff
Medical Research Council's Molecular Immunopathology Unit, and of the
Department of Pathology, University of Cambridge, Cambridge

Deborah Hay

MRCP, FRCPath
Wellcome Trust Clinical Training Fellow
MRC Molecular Haematology Unit
Weatherall Institute of Molecular Medicine, Oxford

David Keeling

MD, FRCP, FRCPath
Consultant Haematologist
Oxford Haemophilia and Thrombosis Centre, Oxford

Ninth Edition

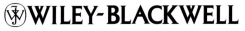

WILEY-BLACKWELL

A John Wiley & Sons, Ltd., Publication

This edition first published 2013 © 2013 by John Wiley & Sons, Ltd

Wiley-Blackwell is an imprint of John Wiley & Sons, formed by the merger of Wiley's global Scientific, Technical and Medical business with Blackwell Publishing.

Registered office: John Wiley & Sons, Ltd, The Atrium, Southern Gate, Chichester, West Sussex, PO19 8SQ, UK

Editorial offices: 9600 Garsington Road, Oxford, OX4 2DQ, UK
The Atrium, Southern Gate, Chichester, West Sussex, PO19 8SQ, UK
111 River Street, Hoboken, NJ 07030-5774, USA

For details of our global editorial offices, for customer services and for information about how to apply for permission to reuse the copyright material in this book please see our website at www.wiley.com/wiley-blackwell.

Library of Congress Cataloging-in-Publication Data

Lecture notes. Haematology / Nevin C. Hughes-Jones ... [et al.]. — 9th ed.
    p. ; cm.
    Haematology
    Rev. ed. of: Lecture notes. Haematology / N.C. Hughes-Jones, S.N. Wickramasinghe, C.S.R. Hatton. 8th ed. 2009.
    Includes bibliographical references and index.
    ISBN 978-0-470-67359-1 (pbk. : alk. paper)
    I. Hughes-Jones, N. C. (Nevin Campbell)   II. Title: Haematology.
    [DNLM: 1. Hematologic Diseases.   2. Blood Physiological Processes. WH 120]
    616.1'5—dc23

                                                                                    2012031978

A catalogue record for this book is available from the British Library.

Wiley also publishes its books in a variety of electronic formats. Some content that appears in print may not be available in electronic books.

Cover image: iStock © Activ Design
Cover design by Grounded Design

Set in 8.5/11pt Utopia Std by Aptara® Inc., New Delhi, India
Printed and bound in Malaysia by Vivar Printing Sdn Bhd

1   2013

Contents

Companion website

This book is accompanied by a companion website:

www.lecturenoteseries.com/haematology

The website includes:

- Key revision points for each chapter in both PowerPoint and PDF format
- Interactive multiple choice questions for each chapter
- Figures from the book in PowerPoint format

Preface to the first edition

These lecture notes are designed to supply the basic knowledge of both the clinical and laboratory aspects of haematological diseases and blood transfusion. The content is broadly similar to that of the course given to medical students by the Department of Haematology at St. Mary's Hospital Medical School. References have been cited so that those who need to extend their knowledge in any particular field can do so. Most of the journals and books that are mentioned are those commonly found in every library.

At the end of each chapter I have supplied learning objectives in studying each disease. There are two main purposes in these objectives. First, they facilitate the learning process, since the process of acquisition, retention, and recall of data is greatly helped if the facts and concepts are centred around a particular objective. Secondly, many objectives are closely related to the practical problems encountered in the diagnosis and treatment of patients. For instance, the following objectives: "to understand the method of differentiation of megaloblastic anaemia due to vitamin B12 deficiency from that due to folate deficiency" and "to understand the basis for the differentiation of leukaemia into acute and chronic forms based on the clinical picture and on the peripheral blood findings" are practical problems encountered frequently in the haematology laboratory. A point of more immediate interest to the undergraduate is that examiners setting either multiple choice or essay questions will be searching for the same knowledge that is required in answering the objectives.

I should like to thank Prof. P.L. Mollison, Dr. P. Barkhan, Dr. I. Chanarin, Dr. G.J. Jenkins, and Dr. M.S. Rose for their criticism and helpful suggestions during the preparation of the manuscript and Mrs. Inge Barnett for typing the several drafts and final typescript.

N.C. Hughes-Jones

Preface to the ninth edition

The science and practice of haematology continue to advance at an extraordinary rate. At the same time, the volume of data that medical students are required to assimilate across all disciplines continues to expand. Therefore, our aim in revising the text of *Lecture Notes in Haematology* was to provide a comprehensive overview of this diverse subject in a way that promotes understanding of pathophysiological concepts, while highlighting the most up-to-date aspects of clinical practice. Further, to enhance active learning, we have also provided a companion website with self-test multiple-choice questions and explanations.

Dr Sunil Wickramasinghe was actively involved in *Lecture Notes* from its inception in the 1970s until the eighth edition. His tragically premature death in 2009 deprives us of a senior author and highly valued colleague. His contribution has been greatly missed.

We have been fortunate in having the help of many of our clinical colleagues for this edition: special thanks are due to Dr Karthik Ramasamy and Dr Adam Mead, both of Oxford University Hospitals, for kindly reviewing the chapters on myeloma and myeloid malignancies respectively. As in previous editions, we also express our thanks to Professor Kevin Gatter of the Nuffield Department of Clinical and Laboratory Sciences, University of Oxford, for generously providing many of the photomicrographs used in this text.

As ever, we are grateful to readers who have taken the time to give us valuable feedback on earlier editions. We hope that the ninth edition of *Haematology Lecture Notes* provides a useful introduction to this fascinating area of medicine.

Chris S. R. Hatton
Nevin C. Hughes-Jones
Deborah Hay
David Keeling

An introduction to haematopoiesis

Learning objectives

✓ To understand the process of formation of blood cells

✓ To understand the concept of a stem cell

✓ To appreciate the process of lineage specification of blood cells

✓ To recognize the different types of mature blood cell

✓ To understand the normal role of each mature cell type in the blood

Where is blood formed?

Blood is normally formed early in the process of embryogenesis, with haemopoietic stem cells originating in the para-aortic mesoderm of the embryo. Primitive red blood cells, platelet precursors and macrophages are initially formed in the vasculature of the extra-embryonic yolk sac, before the principal site of haemopoiesis shifts to the fetal liver at around five to eight weeks' gestation. The liver remains the main source of blood in the fetus until shortly before birth, although the bone marrow starts to develop haemopoietic activity from as early as 10 weeks' gestation.

After birth, the marrow is the sole site of haemopoiesis in healthy individuals. During the first few years of life, nearly all the marrow cavities contain red haemopoietic marrow, but this recedes such that by adulthood haemopoiesis is limited to marrow in the vertebrae, pelvis, sternum and the proximal ends of the femora and humeri, with minor contributions from the skull bones, ribs and scapulae.

Although the sites of haemopoiesis in the adult are therefore relatively limited, other sites retain their capacity to produce blood cells if needed. In conditions in which there is an increased haemopoietic drive (such as chronic haemolytic anaemias and chronic myeloproliferative disorders), haemopoietic tissue will expand and may extend into marrow cavities that do not normally support haemopoiesis in the adult. Foci of haemopoietic tissue may also appear in the adult liver and spleen (known as extramedullary haemopoiesis).

Haemopoietic stem cells

The process of haemopoiesis involves both the specification of individual blood cell lineages and cellular proliferation to maintain adequate circulating numbers of cells throughout life. This is accomplished using the unique properties of haemopoietic stem cells.

Long-term haemopoietic stem cells (HSCs) in the bone marrow are capable of both self-renewal and differentiation into the progenitors of individual blood cell lineages. The progenitor cells of individual lineages then undergo many rounds of division and further differentiation in order to yield populations of mature blood cells. This process can be represented as a hierarchy of cells, with HSCs giving rise to populations of precursor cells, which in turn give rise to cells increasingly committed to producing a single type of mature blood cell (Figure 1.1). Thus, the immediate progeny of HSCs are the multipotent progenitor cells, which have limited self-renewal capacity but retain

Haematology Lecture Notes, Ninth edition. C.S.R. Hatton, N.C. Hughes-Jones, D. Hay and D. Keeling. © 2013 John Wiley & Sons, Ltd.
Published 2013 by John Wiley & Sons, Ltd.

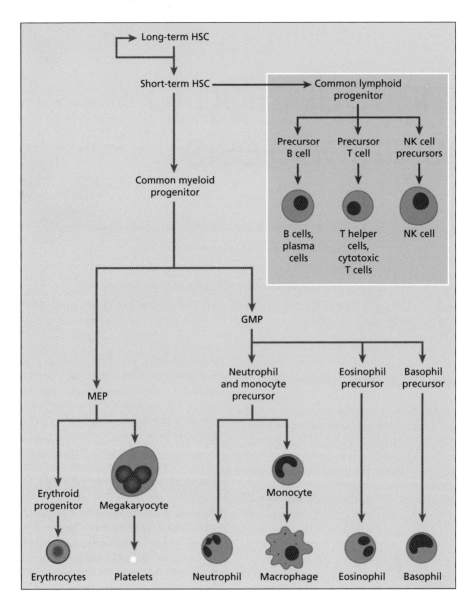

Figure 1.1 A schematic representation of the process of haemopoiesis. Multipotent stem cells give rise to lymphoid (pink) and myeloid (blue) lineages. The myeloid lineage further divides into granulocytic, erythroid and megakaryocytic (platelet) lineages. As cells progress through this process of differentiation, they accrue more functional specialization and lose their multipotency.
Abbreviations: HSC – haemopoietic stem cell; MEP – megakaryocyte/erythroid progenitor; GMP – granulocyte macrophage progenitor; NK – natural killer

the ability to differentiate into all blood cell lineages. Although there is still debate about exactly how lineage restricted subsequent precursors are, the concept of sequential and irreversible differentiation is widely accepted. In Figure 1.1, the HSC is seen giving rise to two major lineages: the lymphoid lineage, in which a common lymphoid progenitor gives rise to B and T cells; and a myeloid lineage, with a common myeloid progenitor giving rise to red cells, granulocytes and platelets. The division of haemopoiesis into myeloid and lymphoid compartments is fundamental to an understanding of haematological disease.

The process of haemopoiesis outlined above has several advantages. First, it permits the massive expansion of cell numbers needed to maintain an adequate population of mature blood cells. It also means that the production of each type of mature blood cell can be controlled individually, tailoring production to specific physiological requirements. Finally it requires relatively little proliferative activity on the part of the long-term HSCs themselves, thereby minimizing the risk of developing mutations in these crucial cells during DNA replication and cell division.

HSCs were first detected and defined functionally through experiments in which a subset of cells from the bone marrow were shown to produce blood cells of all lineages when transplanted into lethally irradiated mice, which have no haemopoietic potential of their own. Subsequent work has used cell surface markers and flow cytometric techniques (see Chapter 5) to define this population: positivity for the cell surface marker CD34 combined with negativity for CD38 describes a population of cells that is also capable of regenerating all cell lineages from the bone marrow. The cell surface marker CD34 is also used to isolate cells with multipotency and self-renewal capacity for stem cell transplantation.

Differentiating blood cells

Precisely how the ultimate lineage choice of differentiating progenitor cells is determined remains a subject of research. It has been argued that factors intrinsic to the HSC itself, such as stochastic fluctuations in transcription factors, may direct lineage specification. However, it is also known that proper regulation of HSCs and progenitor cells requires their interaction with extrinsic factors, such as non-haemopoietic cells in the bone marrow niche (e.g. endothelial cells and osteoblastic progenitors). HSCs and progenitor cells are not randomly distributed in the marrow, but exist in ordered proximity relative to mesenchymal cells, endothelial cells and the vasculature. Signalling from these non-haemopoietic cells, plus physiochemical cues such as hypoxia and blood flow, are therefore likely to influence the transcriptional activity and fate of HSCs.

Myelopoiesis

Signalling through myeloid growth factors such as granulocyte-macrophage colony stimulating factor (GM-CSF) is essential for the survival and proliferation of myeloid cells. The specification of the myeloid lineage is also known to require the interaction of a series of specific transcription factors, including C/EBPα, Core

Binding Factor and c-Myb. As well as being essential for the normal formation of myeloid cells, it is becoming clear that an appreciation of these factors and others like them is critical for an understanding of myeloid diseases such as acute myeloid leukaemia (see Chapter 11).

The separation of the erythroid and megakaryocytic components of myelopoiesis requires the action of transcription factors GATA1, NF-E2 and SCL, and signalling through the growth factors thrombopoietin and erythropoietin.

Granulocytes and their function

Morphologically, myeloblasts are the earliest recognizable granulocytic cells. They are large cells, with open nuclear chromatin (Figure 1.2(a)). The successive stages through which a myeloblast matures into circulating neutrophil granulocytes are termed promyelocytes (Figure 1.2(b)), neutrophil myelocytes (Figure 1.2(c)), neutrophil metamyelocytes and neutrophil band cells. Cell division occurs in myeloblasts, promyelocytes and myelocytes, but not normally in metamyelocytes and band cells.

The maturation process of the neutrophil lineage is characterized by a reduction in size of the cell, along with the acquisition of granules containing agents essential for their microbicidal function. The nucleus also gradually begins to adopt its characteristic segmented shape (Figure 1.3).

Mature neutrophils have the ability to migrate to areas of inflammation (chemotaxis), where they become marginated in the vessel lumen and pass into the tissues through interaction with selectins, integrins and other cell adhesion molecules. Once primed by cytokines such as TNFα and IFNγ, neutrophils are able to phagocytose opsonized microbes, and destroy them by deploying their toxic intracellular contents. This release of reactive oxygen species (the 'respiratory burst') provides a substrate for the enzyme myeloperoxidase (MPO), which then generates hypochlorous acid with direct cytotoxic effects. The granules of neutrophils also contain an array of antimicrobial agents, including defensins, chymotrypsin and gelatinases.

Eosinophils (a subset of granulocytes with bright pink granules on haematoxylin and eosin-stained blood films) have a similar ability to phagocytose and destroy micro-organisms, but are classically associated with the immune response to parasitic infection. They are often found in high numbers in patients with allergy and atopy. IL-5 signalling appears to be critical for their differentiation from granulocyte precursors.

Basophils are the least common of the granulocytes. They contain very prominent cytoplasmic

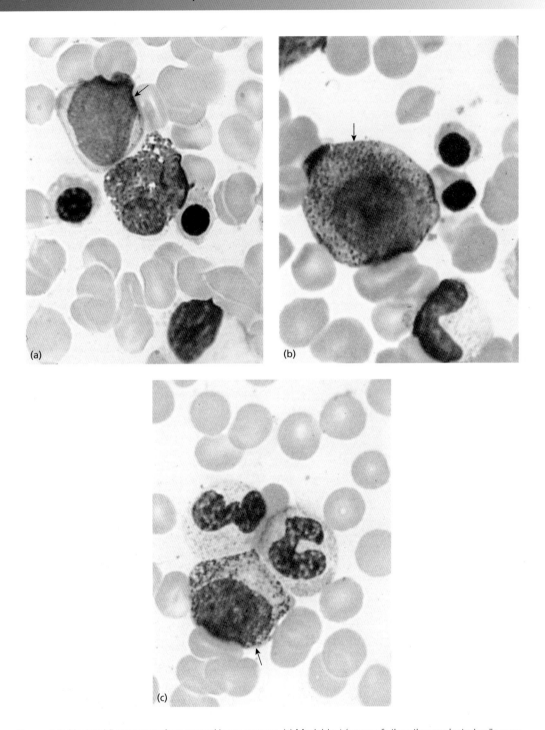

(a)

(b)

(c)

Figure 1.2 Neutrophil precursors from normal bone marrow. (a) Myeloblast (arrowed); the other nucleated cells near the myeloblast are an eosinophil granulocyte (centre) and two polychromatic erythroblasts. (b) Promyelocyte (arrowed); the other nucleated cells are two polychromatic erythroblasts and a neutrophil metamyelocyte. (c) Neutrophil myelocyte (arrowed); there are two neutrophil band cells adjacent to the myelocyte.

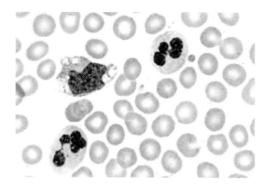

Figure 1.3 Monocyte and two neutrophil granulocytes – the monocyte has a pale, greyish-blue vacuolated cytoplasm.

granules on H&E staining, which have stores of histamine and heparin as well as proteolytic enzymes. They are involved in a variety of immune and inflammatory responses, but it is unusual to see a marked elevation or depression in their numbers in specific reactive conditions.

Monocytopoiesis and monocyte function

The cell classes belonging to the monocyte–macrophage lineage are, in increasing order of maturity, monoblasts, promonocytes, marrow monocytes, blood monocytes and tissue macrophages. Their synthesis is controlled in part by the activity of GM-CSF. Functionally, monocytes have a variety of immune roles: as the precursors of tissue macrophages and dendritic cells, their roles include phagocytosis, antibody presentation to other immune cells, and a contribution to the cytokine milieu. Phagocytosis of micro-organisms and cells coated with antibody (with their exposed Fc fragments) and complement occurs via binding to Fc and C3b receptors on the surface of monocytes and macrophages. Bacteria and fungi that are not antibody coated are phagocytosed after binding to mannose receptors on the phagocyte surface. As with neutrophils, the killing of phagocytosed micro-organisms by monocytes/macrophages involves superoxide dependent and O_2- independent mechanisms.

Megakaryocytes and platelet function

Megakaryocytes are the cells which give rise to platelets. During megakaryocyte formation, driven by the action of the growth factor thrombopoietin (TPO), there is replication of DNA without cell division. This leads to the generation of very large mononucleate cells that are markedly polyploid. A mature megakaryocyte is illustrated in Figure 1.4. Large numbers of platelets are formed from the cytoplasm of each mature megakaryocyte; these are rapidly discharged directly into the marrow sinusoids. The residual 'bare' megakaryocyte nucleus is then phagocytosed by macrophages.

TPO is the key regulator of normal platelet production. This protein, which is produced by the liver, binds to TPO receptors on the megakaryocyte membrane. Downstream signalling through mechanisms including the JAK/STAT pathway allows an increase in megakaryocyte ploidy, and also cytoplasmic maturation such that increased numbers of platelets are released. TPO is also able to bind to the surface of platelets themselves; thus when platelet numbers are high, TPO is sequestered on the platelet membranes, leaving less available to act on the megakaryocytes to promote further platelet production. In this way, a negative feedback loop is created, maintaining platelet numbers within stable limits.

The fundamental role of platelets is in primary haemostasis, through their interactions with von Willebrand factor and the exposed collagen of damaged endothelial surfaces (see Chapter 14).

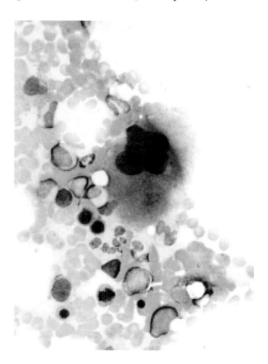

Figure 1.4 Mature megakaryocyte (centre). This is a very large cell with a single lobulated nucleus. Compare the size of the megakaryocyte with that of the other nucleated marrow cells in this figure.

Erythropoiesis and red cell function

The specification of the erythroid lineage requires a balanced interaction between transcription factors GATA1 and other haemopoietic transcription factors, including PU.1 and FOG1. Once committed to an erythroid fate, the expansion of erythroid precursors takes place, driven largely by signalling through the erythropoietin receptor.

The hormone erythropoietin is expressed principally in the cortical interstitial cells of the kidney, where its transcription is modulated in response

to hypoxaemia. The transcription factor *hypoxia inducible factor* (HIF-1) is induced in cells exposed to hypoxaemic conditions enhances expression of the erythropoietin gene. Increased levels of erythropoietin are therefore available to interact with the Epo receptor on red cell progenitor membranes, activating an erythroid-specific signal transduction cascade, and leading to enhanced proliferation and terminal differentiation of erythroid cells.

Morphologically, the differentiation and maturation of erythroid cells are shown in Figure 1.5. Proerythroblasts are early erythroid progenitors in the bone marrow recognizable by their large size, their

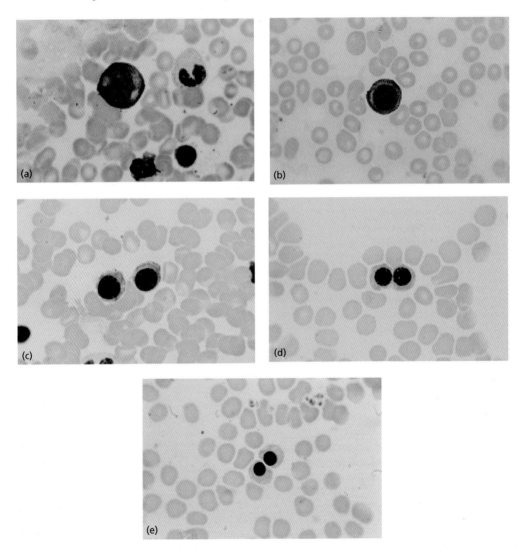

Figure 1.5 (a) Proerythroblast, (b) basophilic normoblast, (c) two early polychromatic normoblasts, (d) two late polychromatic normoblasts and (e) two more mature late polychromatic normoblasts. The condensed chromatin in the basophilic normoblast is slightly coarser than in the proerythroblast. The nuclei of the late polychromatic normoblasts contain large masses of condensed chromatin.

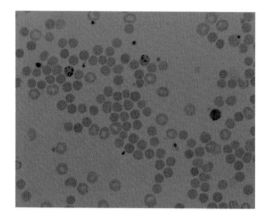

Figure 1.6 Reticulocytes in peripheral blood stained supravitally with brilliant cresyl blue. Note the reticulum of precipitated ribosomes.

dark blue cytoplasm, their dispersed nuclear chromatin and nucleoli. As the cells mature, they become smaller with less basophilic cytoplasm (see Figure 1.5). Cell division continues until the cells reach the late polychromatic normoblast stage, when cells extrude their nucleus. At this point the cell is termed a reticulocyte (Figure 1.6) and is released from the marrow into the peripheral blood. Reticulocytes are characterized by their slightly larger size and bluish staining contrasted with mature red cells. After one to two days in circulation, reticulocytes lose their remaining ribosomes and become mature red cells.

The red cell function is to carry oxygen, bound to the haem moiety of haemoglobin, from the lungs to the peripheral tissues. The details of haemoglobin structure and function (and diseases resulting from perturbation of these) are discussed further in Chapter 4.

Lymphopoiesis

The structure and function of lymphoid tissue are the focus of Chapter 6. Lymphoid cells are thought to arise from multilymphoid progenitor cells in the fetal marrow. Although incompletely characterized, these progenitors are known to feature CD45 and CD7 cell surface markers. The transcription factor Ikaros has been shown to be critical for lymphopoiesis in mouse models; Pax5 is among several transcription factors needed for B cell development, while GATA3 and Notch signalling are essential for T cell maturation.

The development of B lymphocytes commences in the fetal liver and fetal marrow. Here, progenitor B cells develop into pre-B cells (defined by the presence of the cytoplasmic μ chain of the B-cell receptor) and then into mature B cells. During this time, the genes for the immunoglobulin light and heavy chains are rearranged, allowing the production of immunoglobulins with a wide array of antigenic specificities. Subsequent B cell maturation requires antigen exposure in the lymph nodes and other secondary lymphoid tissues, with the mature B cell having the capacity to recognize non-self antigens and produce large quantities of specific immunoglobulin.

T cells, by contrast, are formed in the thymus, where lymphocyte progenitors from the fetal liver migrate in early gestation. These earliest immature T cells express neither CD4 nor CD8 and undergo rearrangement of the T cell receptor genes to permit cell surface expression of the T cell receptor (TCR). As with the surface immunoglobulin or B cell receptor, the process of rearrangement yields a vast collection of potential T cell receptors, with the ability to recognize a wide range of different antigens. During the process of maturation, T cells acquire both CD4 and CD8 cell surface markers (double positive thymocytes) and undergo a process of positive selection to ensure that the survival only of those that are able to interact adequately with MHC molecules on antigen-presenting cells. T cells that interact with MHC Class I become CD8 positive only, while those that interact with MHC class II down-regulate their CD8 expression and become CD4 T cells. A further phase of negative selection ensures that T cells that interact very strongly with 'self-antigens' in the thymus undergo apoptosis.

CD4+ lymphocytes are known as T 'helper' cells, and they form the majority of the circulating T cell population. Their roles include the production of cytokines to promote an inflammatory response in presence of the appropriate antigen. Such cytokines include interferon γ (from the Th1 class of CD4+ cells) and interleukins 4, 5 and 13 (from the Th2 subset of CD4+ cells). The effects of cytokine production include activation of the monocyte/macrophage system, the promotion of granulocyte maturation and the induction of antibody synthesis by B cells.

CD8+ lymphocytes are T suppressor/cytotoxic cells, comprising approximately one quarter of the T cells in the peripheral blood. Their function is to destroy any cells expressing a peptide to which their T cell receptor can bind (e.g. virally infected cells).

A small minority of mature lymphocytes are distinct from both B and T cell lineages. These are the natural

Table 1.1 The sequence of events during B-cell differentiation.

Characteristic	Pre-pre-B cell	Pre-B cell	Immature B cell	Mature B cell	Plasma cell
Heavy-chain genes rearranged	+	+	+	+	+
Light-chain genes rearranged	−/+	+	+	+	+
Terminal deoxynucleotidyl-transferase	+	+/−	−	−	−
Cytoplasmic μ-chains expressed	−	+	−	−	−
Surface IgM (but not IgD) expressed	−	−	+	−	−
Surface IgM and IgD expressed	−	−	−	+	−
Cytoplasmic Ig expressed	−	−	−	−	+
CD10	+	+	−	−	−
CD19 and CD20	+	+	+	+	+

killer (NK) cells, which have a role in the innate immune system, through cell-mediated cytotoxicity.

All these stages of both B and T cell development have the morphological features of either lymphoblasts or lymphocytes. The identification of different lymphocyte precursors is therefore based not on morphology but on properties including reactivity with certain monoclonal antibodies, their immunoglobulin gene or TCR gene rearrangement status, and the presence of immunoglobulin or TCR on the surface membrane (Tables 1.1 and 1.2). In the peripheral blood, lymphocytes may be small and compact (Figure 1.7) or may appear large with azurophilic cytoplasmic granules (Figure 1.8). Such large granular lymphocytes include cytotoxic T cells and NK cells.

Table 1.2 The sequence of events during T-cell differentiation.

Characteristic	Pre-T cell	Early thymocyte	Intermediate thymocyte	Late thymocyte	Mature T cell
CD7	+	+	+	+	+
Terminal deoxynucleotidyl-transferase	−/+	+	+	−	−
TCR γ genes rearranged/deleted	−	+	+	+	+
TCR β genes rearranged	−	−	+	+	+
TCR α genes rearranged	−	−	−/+	+	+
CD2	−	+	+	+	+
CD3	−	+	+	+	+
CD4 and CD8	−	−	−/+	−	−
CD4 or CD8	−	−	−	+	+

Note: TCR — T-cell receptor.

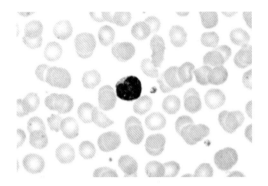

Figure 1.7 A small lymphocyte in a normal blood smear.

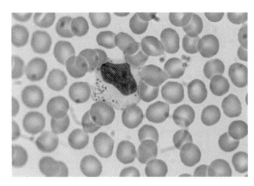

Figure 1.8 A large lymphocyte with several azurophilic cytoplasmic granules. Large granular lymphocytes include cytotoxic T cells and natural killer (NK) cells. *Source*: Courtesy of Dr Barbara Bain.

Summary

Table 1.3 summarizes the role of each mature cell type in the peripheral blood. It is the abnormal production, function or destruction of these cells that constitutes the study of clinical haematology, and that forms the basis of the rest of this text.

Table 1.3 **The main functions of blood cells.**

Type of cell	Main functions
Red blood cells (erythrocytes)	Transport O_2 from lungs to tissues (see Chapters 2 and 4)
Neutrophil granulocytes	Chemotaxis, phagocytosis, killing of phagocytosed bacteria
Eosinophil granulocytes	All neutrophil functions listed above, effector cells for antibody-dependent damage to metazoal parasites, regulate immediate-type hypersensitivity reactions (inactivate histamine and leukotrienes released by basophils and mast cells)
Basophil granulocytes	Mediate immediate-type hypersensitivity (IgE-coated basophils react with specific antigen and release histamine and leukotrienes), modulate inflammatory responses by releasing heparin and proteases
Monocytes and macrophages	Chemotaxis, phagocytosis, killing of some micro-organisms, antigen presentation, release of IL-1 and TNF that stimulate bone marrow stromal cells to produce GM-CSF, G-CSF, M-CSF and IL-6
Platelets	Adhere to subendothelial connective tissue, participate in primary haemostasis
Lymphocytes	Critical for immune responses and production of haemopoietic growth factors

2

Anaemia: General principles

Learning objectives

- ✓ To understand the normal control of red cell production
- ✓ To understand the mechanisms by which anaemia may arise
- ✓ To appreciate the signs and symptoms of anaemia
- ✓ To understand how anaemia can be classified by reticulocyte response and/or by red cell size
- ✓ To be able to suggest causes of microcytic, normocytic and macrocytic anaemia
- ✓ To understand normal iron metabolism, how iron deficiency may arise and how to investigate it
- ✓ To be able to describe how iron overload occurs
- ✓ To understand the pathophysiology and typical laboratory features of the anaemia of chronic disease
- ✓ To understand the normal metabolism of vitamin B12 and folic acid, and to appreciate how megaloblastic anaemia may arise
- ✓ To suggest some normoblastic causes of macrocytosis
- ✓ To appreciate that failure of the normal control of red cell production can lead to polycythaemia

Anaemia

Anaemia is defined as a haemoglobin (Hb) concentration below the reference range for the age and sex of an individual. It is important to recognize that a 'normal' haemoglobin level will be different in individuals of different ages and sexes (Table 2.1). Newborns will have an average Hb of around 17g/dl, which rises over the 24 hours following birth; children tend to have lower normal haemoglobin levels than adults; and women usually have a lower average haemoglobin than men – an effect attributable to the effect of androgens in males. In addition, physiological changes such as pregnancy will also have a predictable effect on haemoglobin concentration and should be taken into account when interpreting the full blood count.

Symptoms and signs of anaemia

When anaemia develops slowly, the associated symptoms are often very mild, since the body has time to adapt to the fall in haemoglobin. This involves mechanisms such as an increase in red cell 2,3-diphosphoglycerate (2,3-DPG), which shifts

Haematology Lecture Notes, Ninth edition. C.S.R. Hatton, N.C. Hughes-Jones, D. Hay and D. Keeling. © 2013 John Wiley & Sons, Ltd.
Published 2013 by John Wiley & Sons, Ltd.

Table 2.1 Reference ranges for Hb values.

	Hb concentration (g/dL)
Cord blood	13.5–20.5
First day of life	15.0–23.5
Children, 6 months–6 years	11.0–14.5
Children, 6–14 years	12.0–15.5
Adult males	13.0–17.0
Adult females (non-pregnant)	12.0–15.5
Pregnant females	11.0–14.0

Table 2.2 Various mechanisms leading to anaemia.

Blood loss

Decreased red cell lifespan (haemolytic anaemia)

    Congenital defect (e.g. sickle cell disease, hereditary spherocytosis)

    Acquired defect (e.g. malaria, some drugs)

Impairment of red cell formation

    Insufficient erythropoiesis

    Ineffective erythropoiesis

Pooling and destruction of red cells in an enlarged spleen

Increased plasma volume (splenomegaly, pregnancy)

the oxygen dissociation curve to the right and permits enhanced delivery of O_2 in the tissues (see Chapter 4). Cardiovascular adaptive mechanisms are also deployed, in the form of increased stroke volume and heart rate. This situation contrasts with that seen in acute-onset anaemia, where the lack of physiological adaptation leads to more marked symptoms and signs at a given haemoglobin level. Significant symptoms may also develop at higher Hb levels in older patients with impaired cardiovascular reserves.

Symptoms of anaemia include lassitude, fatigue, dyspnoea on exertion, palpitations and headache; older patients with impaired cardiovascular reserve may also develop angina and intermittent claudication. Physical signs include pallor, tachycardia, a wide pulse pressure, flow murmurs and, in severe cases, congestive cardiac failure.

The underlying cause of anaemia should always be sought: anaemia is not a final diagnosis in itself, but rather a potential manifestation of a multiplicity of disease states. The physical signs and symptoms of anaemia must therefore be carefully reviewed for clues to its underlying aetiology.

The normal control of red cell production

In healthy adults, there is a steady-state equilibrium between the rate of release of new red cells from the bone marrow into the circulation and the removal of senescent red cells from the circulation by macrophages. The renally secreted hormone erythropoietin (epo) is the main agent responsible for translating tissue hypoxia into increased red cell production to maintain this balance (see also Chapter 1).

For anaemia to arise, there must be either a failure of adequate production of red cells (e.g. insufficient erythroid tissue in the marrow or poor-quality erythroid maturation – see Table 2.2) or an increased rate of red cell loss (perhaps through blood loss or haemolysis). The reticulocyte count is a useful marker to enable differentiation of anaemia due to failure of production from that due to accelerated red cell destruction. Where there is sufficient bone marrow reserve to mount a good response to anaemia, the reticulocyte count will be high. Bone marrow failure syndromes, by contrast, will have a low reticulocyte count. However, in many cases of anaemia, both mechanisms have a role to play: in anaemia due to chronic bleeding from the gastrointestinal tract, for example, red cells are lost from the circulation, while the development of iron deficiency prevents an adequate bone marrow response. Similarly, chronic haemolytic conditions, which are typically associated with a reticulocytosis, may be complicated by the development of folate deficiency; this will impede the bone marrow response and thus limit any reticulocytosis. Thus, although the reticulocyte count is an important part of the assessment of any patient with anaemia, it may not be straightforward to interpret.

Morphological classification of anaemias

An alternative and very widely used strategy for thinking about anaemia is to classify it in terms of red cell size. Characteristic changes in the size of red cells,

Table 2.3 Morphological classification of anaemia.

Type	MCV	Causes
Microcytic and hypochromic, or microcytic	Low	Iron deficiency, thalassaemia syndromes, some cases of anaemia of chronic disorders
Normocytic and normochromic	Normal	Acute blood loss, some cases of anaemia of chronic disorders, chronic renal failure, some haemolytic anaemias, leucoerythroblastic anaemias
Macrocytic	High	Alcoholism, folate deficiency, vitamin B12 deficiency

Notes: MCV — mean cell volume.

and their degree of haemoglobinization, accompany the development of anaemia of different aetiologies, and can be used to divided anaemia into three main groups:

1 Microcytic hypochromic (low mean cell volume and low mean cell haemoglobin).
2 Macrocytic (high mean cell volume).
3 Normocytic (normal mean cell volume).

Thus anaemia due to iron deficiency is typically microcytic and hypochromic, due the failure of adequate haemoglobin production by the red cell. The thalassaemias are also typically microcytic, hypochromic anaemias. By contrast, anaemia due to vitamin B12 or folate deficiency, in which there is a failure of nuclear maturation, is classically macrocytic. Haemolytic anaemias characterized by a brisk reticulocytosis may also have a slightly higher mean cell volume, since reticulocytes tend to be larger than mature red cells. Normocytic anaemias include those due to acute blood loss, where there has not been time to produce a significant marrow response.

The morphological classification of anaemia is not perfect. Some conditions can straddle two categories: the anaemia of chronic disease, which is typically normocytic, but may be slightly microcytic, is a good example. Similarly, anaemia with two contributing mechanisms may produce results that are harder to interpret: in coeliac disease, for instance, there may be a combined deficiency of iron and folic acid, with each blunting the other's effect on the mean cell volume to produce a normocytic anaemia. Nevertheless, the classification of anaemia by mean cell volume does have the merit of highlighting the most frequently seen and readily treated causes of anaemia: namely, haematinic deficiency.

Table 2.3 summarizes the classification of anaemia by mean cell volume and mean cell haemoglobin, and Table 2.4 shows the normal ranges for these indices. A more detailed discussion of the commonest

Table 2.4 Reference ranges for red cell indices in adults.

Index	Normal range
Mean cell volume* (MCV)	82–99 fL
Mean cell Hb (MCH)	27–33 pg
Mean cell Hb concentration (MCHC)	32–36 g/dL

Note: *Lower limit may be as low as 70–74 fL between 1 and 8 years of age, in the absence of iron deficiency.

causes is found in the following sections, and Figure 2.1 shows the classical appearances of red cells in cases of anaemia.

Microcytic anaemia: Iron handling and iron deficiency anaemia

Iron deficiency anaemia is thought to be the commonest cause of anaemia worldwide. An understanding of how it arises and how it can be diagnosed and best treated requires some appreciation of normal iron metabolism, which is outlined below. The consequences of deranged iron absorption and iron overload are also described (see Box 2.1).

Iron absorption

Excess iron is potentially toxic. Therefore, since the body has no physiological mechanism for upregulating iron excretion, very tight controls exist over its absorption from the gut. This permits iron absorption to be maximized when stores are low or when there is a need to increase erythropoiesis, but

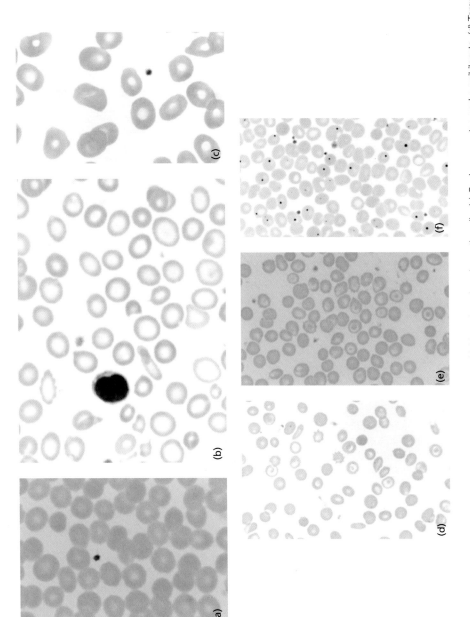

Figure 2.1 Normal and abnormal red cells: (a) Normochromic, normocytic cells. (b) Hypochromic, microcytic cells. (c) Oval macrocytes and a poikilocyte. (d) Target cells, spherocytes and acanthocytes in a blood film from a splenectomized patient. Acanthocytes are red cells with up to about 10 spicules of varying length irregularly distributed over their surface. They are found not only post splenectomy but also in other conditions such as hypothyroidism and advanced alcohol-related cirrhosis of the liver. (e) Target cells from a patient with obstructive jaundice. (f) Howell–Jolly bodies within red cells, found typically in patients post splenectomy. Figures (a)–(c) are at similar magnification; (d)–(f) are at a lower magnification.

Box 2.1: Iron overload

Iron absorption from a normal diet is inappropriately increased in hereditary haemochromatosis, a collection of conditions in which there are defects in the key proteins responsible for iron regulation. In each case, there is a failure of adequate down-regulation of ferroportin by hepcidin, leading to uncontrolled iron transition from the enterocyte to the circulation. If transferrin's ability to bind iron is saturated, non-transferrin-bound iron is found in the circulation; this form may be taken up by many cell types, including hepatocytes and cardiac myocytes, where it has a damaging oxidant effect.

The commonest form is HFE haemochromatosis, an autosomal recessive condition with an incidence of 5 per 1000 in northern European populations. Most patients have a point mutation leading to the amino substitution C282Y; others have compound heterozygosity for C282Y and the H63D mutation. The HFE gene is thought to have a key role in the control of hepatic synthesis of hepcidin, and homozygotes usually develop symptoms from tissue damage due to severe iron overload between the ages of 40 and 60 years. Iron deposition occurs in a variety of organs, leading to cardiac dysfunction, cirrhosis, diabetes mellitus, testicular atrophy and 'bronze' skin pigmentation. Women typically have a rather later age onset of symptoms, due to the protective effect of menstrual iron loss. Other forms of hereditary haemochromatosis exist, due to mutations affecting the ferroportin gene and the transferrin receptor gene, but are much less common.

Iron loading will also occur when there are conflicting signals regarding the body's iron requirements. Consider patients with thalassaemia (see Chapter 4) in whom iron stores are not reduced, but in whom ineffective erythropoiesis leads to a persistent erythroid signal to increase iron absorption. Excess iron absorption from the GI tract in these patients is compounded by iron entering the body through transfusions, and severe iron loading can result.

Whatever the cause, estimations of the extent of iron loading can be made from the serum ferritin, though liver biopsy may be needed to quantify iron levels accurately and assess the extent of hepatic damage. T2* MRI is an excellent method for assessing cardiac iron loading.

Where possible, treatment is by venesection. However, venesection is clearly inappropriate in patients who develop iron overload due to ineffective erythropoiesis and chronic transfusion programmes. Here the use of iron chelators is needed (see also Chapter 4).

---

ensures that there is no excess iron absorbed when stores are good.

The normal Western diet contains 10–20mg of iron per day and typically 5–10% of this is absorbed. Normally, iron in the duodenum is reduced to its ferrous (Fe^{2+}) form by duodenal cytochrome b, before binding the divalent metal transporter DMT1 on the apical (luminal) membrane of the duodenal enterocyte. Iron thus taken up into the cell is either stored directly as ferritin (which may be lost with desquamation of the enterocyte from the lumen of the gut) or oxidized to the ferric form by the transmembrane protein hephaestin and transported to the plasma via the molecule ferroportin on the basolateral membrane of the enterocyte. Iron in the plasma is bound to the transport protein transferrin, which delivers iron to the bone marrow for erythropoiesis. Here it enters the erythroid cells by interacting with the surface transferrin receptor 1. Red cells at the end of their lifespan are removed from the circulation by reticuloendothelial macrophages and have their haem moiety recycled. The iron is released from the haem ring and bound to transferrin to be redelivered to the bone marrow, or stored as ferritin. This process is summarized in Figure 2.2.

Several checkpoints operate during this process. The uptake of iron into the duodenal enterocyte may be affected by the local oxygen tension – mediated by the effect of the transcription factor hypoxia inducible factor (HIF) on the expression of DMT1. The production of DMT1 is also influenced directly by iron: iron affects the binding of iron-response proteins to iron-response elements in the 5′ untranslated region of the mRNA for this gene, determining the rate of its translation.

Once iron is inside the enterocyte, its transfer to the circulation is controlled by the hormone hepcidin. This protein, produced by the liver, binds to ferroportin and induces its internalisation. This prevents the efflux of iron from the enterocyte, such that it will be lost when the cell is desquamated into the lumen of the gut.

Hepcidin expression is itself regulated directly by several mechanisms relevant to the assessment of iron stores. When carrying iron, transferrin is involved in a signalling pathway that enhances hepcidin expression, thus reducing iron absorption from

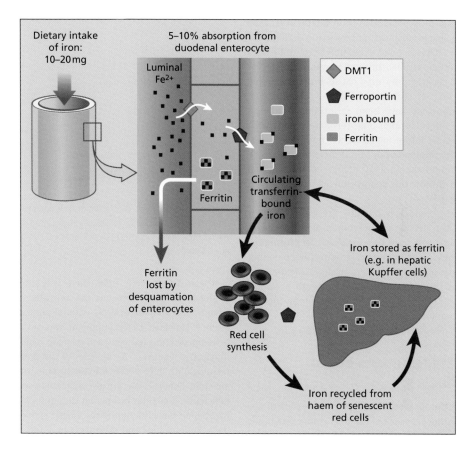

Figure 2.2 A summary of iron handling. Note that there is no physiological mechanism to enhance iron loss after it is absorbed from the duodenal enterocytes. Hepcidin, produced by the liver when iron replete, influences the production and/or function of key molecules in iron absorption, including ferroportin, DMT1 and transferrin.

the gut. By contrast, the hypoxia inducible factor is able to contribute to a decrease in hepcidin expression, as can enhanced erythropoietic activity. In these two circumstances, a reduction in hepcidin will result in increased iron absorption in settings in which additional iron absorption is likely to be beneficial.

In short, although adults who have normal iron stores absorb approximately 5–10% of their total intake (0.5–2 mg/day), this is subject to great variation in response to physiological demand. Hepcidin is the master regulator of this process. In the setting of iron loading, hepcidin expression is up-regulated and iron absorption is limited; where there is a requirement for increased erythroid activity, hepcidin levels fall and more iron absorption is permitted. Clearly, there are situations in which these signals conflict with each other – for example in the thalassaemias, when anaemia and iron loading coexist (see Box 2.1 and Chapter 4). Here, pharmacological means of iron control must be employed.

How does iron deficiency arise?

Iron deficiency will arise in any of three settings:

1 A diet containing too little iron to meet physiological needs.
2 Malabsorption of iron from the duodenum.
3 Increased loss of iron, e.g. through haemorrhage.

Iron deficiency is not uncommon in infants who are given unsupplemented milk or who are exclusively breast fed for more than six months. Similarly, the increased iron requirements of growing children and menstruating women can also put them at risk of dietary iron deficiency. As the physiological requirements for iron rise substantially during pregnancy, iron deficiency is common here, even in the context of a good diet. Iron is most readily absorbed in its haem form, as non-haem iron may be bound by phytates and phosphates also found in food. Vegan diets, containing principally non-haem iron, may therefore also predispose to dietary iron deficiency.

Gastric HCl is needed to reduce ferric to ferrous iron for efficient absorption. Therefore partial or complete gastrectomy may cause iron deficiency through lack of HCl (achlorhydria). Certain ant-acid compounds have been described as having a similar effect, though long-term treatment with proton-pump inhibitors such as omeprazole appears to be implicated in iron deficiency only very rarely. Duodenal pathology such as coeliac disease may also inhibit the absorption of iron from an adequate diet.

However, blood loss remains the most frequent cause of iron deficiency. In women of childbearing age, menorrhagia must be considered; in postmenopausal women and in men, gastrointestinal bleeding is the most likely explanation, and an unexplained finding of iron deficiency should prompt a careful evaluation for gastric and colonic pathology, including malignancies.

These causes are summarized in Table 2.5.

The manifestations of iron deficiency

Although iron is found in every cell (as part of co-factors for the enzymes of the respiratory chain, for instance), at any time the bulk of iron in a healthy individual is found in red cells. Haematological manifestations are among the first seen in iron deficiency.

Table 2.5 **Causes of iron deficiency.**
Reduced iron stores at birth due to prematurity
Inadequate intake (prolonged breast or bottle feeding without iron supplementation, vegetarian diets, poverty)
Increased requirement (pregnancy and lactation)

Chronic haemorrhage
   Uterine (menorrhagia)
   Gastrointestinal (e.g. peptic ulceration; Meckel's diverticulum; colonic diverticulosis, ulcerative colitis, carcinoma of the stomach, colon or rectum, haemorrhoids, hookworm infestation*)
   Others (e.g. self-inflicted, recurrent haematuria)

Malabsorption (coeliac disease, partial gastrectomy, atrophic gastritis)
Chronic intravascular haemolysis leading to haemoglobinuria and haemosiderinuria (rare)
Note: * This is a very common cause of iron deficiency in tropical countries.

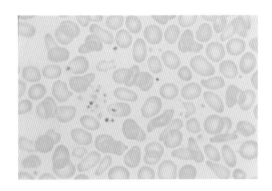

Figure 2.3 Peripheral blood film from a patient with untreated iron deficiency anaemia. Hypochromic microcytes and elongated ('pencil-shaped') poikilocytes are present.

If iron deficiency is mild, there will simply be a depletion of iron stores in the reticuloendothelial system. This may be entirely without clinical consequence. However, as the supply of iron to the tissues is hampered, the red cells will develop hypochromic microcytic features. As deficiency progresses, the haemoglobin falls, giving a hypochromic, microcytic anaemia. Other tissues are also affected in severe iron deficiency: there may be angular stomatitis, brittle and misshapen nails (including the classic spoon-shaped nails, koilonychia) and dysphagia in some cases associated with a pharyngeal stricture or web. Some patients also manifest bizarre dietary cravings, known as pica. With earlier diagnosis, these 'textbook' signs and symptoms are now much less frequently seen.

The blood film will show characteristic features: in addition to the hypochromic, microcytic red cells, there may be misshapen red cells (poikilocytes), including pencil cells and target cells. These are shown in Figure 2.3. The inability of the bone marrow to respond adequately will result in a reticulocyte count lower than expected for the degree of anaemia.

Confirming a diagnosis of iron deficiency

While the combination of a microcytic hypochromic anaemia with a likely history may strongly suggest iron deficiency, confirmation is still required. The key laboratory parameters of iron status are the serum ferritin, transferrin and serum iron levels. While none is a perfect indicator of iron status, all three together permit the best estimation of iron status short of invasive tests like bone marrow biopsy.

Ferritin is the main storage protein for iron and for concentrations <4000μg/L it roughly correlates with

Table 2.6 Measurements of iron status in people with normal iron stores, individuals with iron depletion without anaemia, and in iron deficiency anaemia.

	Normal iron stores	Depleted iron stores		
		Without reduction of iron supply to tissues	Reduced iron supply to tissues, no anaemia	Iron deficiency anaemia
Serum ferritin (µg/L)	20–300	Usually <20	<20	<20
Transferrin (g/L)	1.7–3.4	Sometimes >3.4	>3.4	>3.4
Serum iron (µmol/L)	10–30	Normal	<10	<10
Transferrin saturation (%)	>16	>16	<16	<16
Hb concentration	Normal	Normal	Within reference range	Below reference range

the amount of tissue-storage iron. As might be predicted, ferritin levels are low in iron deficiency (see Table 2.6). However, there is no single value for ferritin concentration that clearly separates individuals with good iron stores from those without, and there is a considerable overlap in ferritin levels between these two groups. In the study illustrated in Figure 2.4, all women with ferritin levels below 14 µg/L were iron deficient; but 25% of the iron-deficient women had ferritin levels above this value. This discrepancy arises because ferritin is also an acute phase reactant, which is typically raised in infection and inflammation. Thus normal serum ferritin levels may be found in the presence of reduced iron stores in acute and chronic infections and in malignancy.

Serum iron also falls in the context of iron deficiency, but there are often marked diurnal and day-to-day changes in serum iron concentration. This, plus recognized reductions in the serum iron concentration in the context of infection and inflammation, make it an unreliable indictor of iron status when assayed alone.

Serum iron can, however, be interpreted in the context of the transferrin concentration, to give a measure of transferrin saturation (iron/transferrin × 100). Transferrin, synthesized in the liver, is generally increased in states of iron deficiency; along with the reduced serum iron, this leads to a reduction in transferrin saturation. A transferrin saturation of <20% generally represents iron depletion, while levels >45% suggest iron loading. However, as with ferritin,

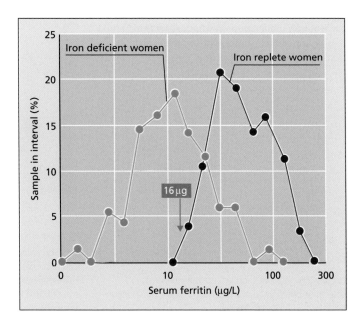

Figure 2.4 The distribution of the serum ferritin concentration in 105 women with stainable iron in the bone marrow (●) and in 69 women with no stainable iron (●). *Source*: From Hallberg *et al.* (1993) *Br. J. Haematol.* **85**, 787–98.

factors other than iron status can have an impact on transferrin levels. Chronic liver disease and chronic inflammatory states will cause the transferrin level to fall, while its production is often increased in women taking the oral contraceptive pill.

A less frequently requested test is estimation of the soluble transferrin receptor concentration. The expression of the transferrin receptor on cells' plasma membranes is regulated by iron availability. Both the transmembrane form and a cleaved soluble form are increased in iron deficiency and in other conditions that give rise to erythroid hyperplasia, but they are not affected in the anaemia of chronic disease.

The gold standard test, undertaken when uncertainty still exists despite testing each of the above, is to stain a bone marrow aspirate with Perls' Prussian Blue stain. This will highlight insoluble iron stores that would be absent in iron deficiency anaemia (compare figures 2.5 and 2.6).

Treating iron deficiency

It is important to address the underlying cause of iron deficiency. If there is gastrointestinal bleeding, its source should be found and treated; malabsorption due to coeliac or Crohn's disease should be controlled. Oral iron supplementation should then be effective, with ferrous sulphate 200mg three times per day being a standard regimen. Continuing this for three months after the normalization of haemoglobin levels will allow replenishment of iron stores. A reticulocytosis is expected in response to treatment, with a rise in the haemoglobin level of 2g/dl over three weeks. For patients who cannot tolerate any form of iron orally, those in whom substantial blood loss continues and those with a severe malabsorption syndrome, parenteral iron preparations exist.

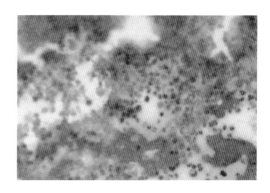

Figure 2.6 Marrow fragment from a patient with iron deficiency anaemia showing an absence of storage iron (Perls' acid ferrocyanide stain). Contrast with Figure 2.5

Iron sucrose (Venofer) and low molecular weight iron dextran (CosmoFer) are both administered intravenously, and the latter may be given as a single total replacement dose by infusion. Adverse effects of intravenous iron therapy include anaphylaxis, fever and arthropathy.

Other causes of microcytic hypochromic anaemia

These are shown in Table 2.2. Thalassaemia is the main differential diagnosis of iron deficiency anaemia. It is discussed in more detail in Chapter 4.

Other causes of microcytic hypochromic anaemia are rare, but include sideroblastic anaemia. Sideroblasts are red cell precursors with a perinuclear ring of coarse iron-containing mitochondria (Figures 2.7 and 2.8).

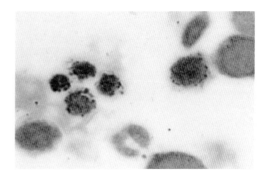

Figure 2.7 Marrow smear from a patient with primary acquired sideroblastic anaemia, stained by the Perls' acid ferrocyanide method (Prussian blue reaction). The erythroblasts contain several coarse blue–black iron-containing granules, which are often arranged around the nucleus.

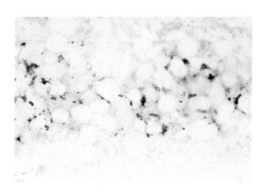

Figure 2.5 Marrow fragment containing normal quantities of storage iron. The haemosiderin stains blue (Perls' acid ferrocyanide stain).

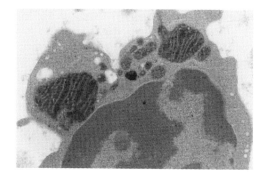

Figure 2.8 Electron micrograph of part of a ring sideroblast showing very electron-dense material between the cristae of enlarged mitochondria.

This condition may be found either as an inherited (usually X-linked) or an acquired form. The common form of X-linked sideroblastic anaemia is caused by mutations in the erythroid-specific δ-aminolaevulinate synthase (ALAS2) gene. ALAS is the enzyme catalysing the first step in haem synthesis. Pyridoxal phosphate is required both for enzyme activity and enzyme stability and some patients with sideroblastic anaemia respond to high doses of pyridoxine given orally. The acquired condition is seen in some cases of myelodysplasia (p. 97) and may also be secondary to excessive alcohol consumption, certain drugs (e.g. isoniazid or chloramphenicol) and lead poisoning.

Normocytic anaemia

The anaemia of chronic disease

The anaemia of chronic disease (ACD) is among the commonest causes of normocytic anaemia. It is associated with chronic inflammatory conditions (e.g. rheumatoid arthritis), chronic infections (e.g. tuberculosis) and malignancies, and its pathogenesis is complex. The activation of macrophages in the underlying chronic condition results in a reduced red cell lifespan, and this is compounded by an insufficient response from the marrow in terms of enhanced erythropoiesis. The signalling through the erythropoietin receptor appears blunted when contrasted to anaemia of other aetiologies, and the response to exogenous erythropoietin is also limited. Furthermore, links between the control of iron handling and inflammatory states are evident from the effect of cytokines such as IL-6 and TNF-α in increasing hepcidin synthesis. As well as limiting iron absorption, the increased hepcidin levels will

also reduce the amount of stored iron released from macrophages and made available for erythropoiesis, since the release of iron from these cells requires ferroportin (the same mechanism needed for the export of iron from enterocytes).

While the red cells in the anaemia of chronic disease are most often normocytic and normochromic, in 30–35% of patients they are hypochromic and microcytic. However, differences in the pattern of iron handling usually help in the distinction between anaemia of chronic disease and iron deficiency. In both conditions, the serum iron concentration is low, but while iron deficiency is characterized by a low serum ferritin and high transferrin, ACD tends to have a normal to high ferritin and low transferrin. If the diagnosis from the peripheral blood tests is still in doubt, the presence or absence of storage iron in the marrow can be determined. Characteristically, iron stores are normal or increased in the anaemia of chronic disorders and absent in iron deficiency anaemia.

Other causes of normocytic anaemia

As shown in Table 2.3, these include acute blood loss; marrow infiltration, for example by malignancy; and the anaemia associated with renal disease, which is due to a reduction in erythropoietin secretion in response to hypoxaemia.

It is important to recognize that many patients will have anaemia with contributions from more than one of these mechanisms. Dissecting the principal reasons for a patient's anaemia may therefore be far from straightforward, and empirical approaches to treatment are sometimes needed.

Macrocytic anaemia

Macrocytic anaemias can be divided into those showing megaloblastic erythropoiesis and those with normoblastic erythropoiesis. Megaloblastic erythropoiesis describes abnormal red cell development characterized by a lack of synchrony between the maturation of the red cell nucleus and its cytoplasm. It arises as a consequence of disordered DNA synthesis and results in a macrocytic anaemia, often with disordered granulocyte and platelet production in addition. Normoblastic erythropoiesis describes the normal appearance of red cell maturation – but may still be associated with a macrocytosis in the peripheral blood. Key causes in both categories are discussed below.

Causes of megaloblastic anaemia: vitamin B12 and folate deficiency

Folic acid is required for several enzymatic reactions in the body, but among the most important is the conversion of deoxyuridylate (dUMP) to deoxythymidylate (dTTP). This is essential for synthesis of thymidine, one of the pyrimidine bases in DNA. Without folic acid, DNA synthesis is hampered (Figure 2.9).

Vitamin B12 (cobalamin) is required for only two enzymatic reactions in the body. In the first, cobalamin is a cofactor for the conversion of methylmalonyl CoA into succinyl CoA, thus allowing the breakdown products of certain amino acids to enter the Krebs cycle. The second reaction is a methyltransferase reaction, which converts homocysteine to methionine (by adding a methyl group) and 5-methyl tetrahydrofolate to tetrahydrofolate (by removing a methyl group). Again, cobalamin is a cofactor. One of

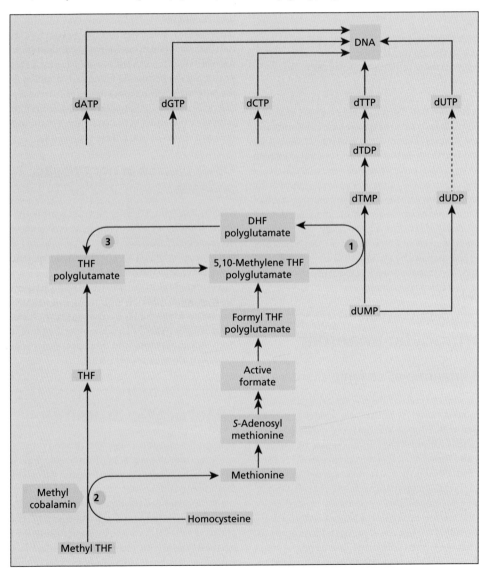

Figure 2.9 Biochemical pathways affected in vitamin B12 and folate deficiency. *Notes*: dTMP – deoxythymidine monophosphate; dTTP – deoxythymidine triphosphate; dUMP – deoxyuridine monophosphate; dUTP – deoxyuridine triphosphate; THF – tetrahydrofolate. Enzymes: 1, thymidylate synthase; 2, homocysteine methyltransferase (methionine synthase); 3, dihydrofolate reductase.

Table 2.7 Key features of vitamin B12 and folate nutrition and absorption.

	Vitamin B12	Folate
Dietary sources	Only foods of animal origin, especially liver	Most foods, especially liver, green vegetables and yeast; destroyed by cooking
Average daily intake[a]	5 μg	400 μg
Minimum daily requirement[a]	1–3 μg	100–200 μg[b]
Body stores[a]	3–5 mg, mainly in the liver	8–20 mg, mainly in the liver
Time to develop deficiency in the absence of intake or absorption[a]	Anaemia in 2–10 years	Macrocytosis in 5 months
Requirements for absorption	Intrinsic factor secreted by gastric parietal cells	Conversion of polyglutamates to monoglutamates by intestinal folate conjugase
Site of absorption	Terminal ileum	Duodenum and jejunum

Notes: [a] In adults. [b] Higher during pregnancy and lactation.

the consequences of vitamin B12 deficiency is a failure to regenerate tetrahydrofolate – and it is this form of folate that is critical for the pyrimidine synthesis step described above.

The consequences of B12 and folate deficiency can therefore be seen to overlap. Both will have a detrimental impact on DNA synthesis, and manifestations of deficiency are seen in the blood where ongoing red cell production is essential.

How do B12 and folate deficiency arise?

Folate is derived from many food sources, both animal and vegetable, with green leafy vegetables providing some of the richest sources (Table 2.7). The Western diet usually contains adequate quantities of folate, though deficiency due to poor intake can be seen especially in frail elderly people and in the context of alcoholism. In some physiological circumstances such as pregnancy and lactation, requirements markedly increase and can result in deficiency; similarly, some disease states can have a similar effect (through an increase in red cell production in chronic haemolytic states, or increased desquamation in psoriasis, for example). Absorption is principally from the duodenum and jejunum; coeliac disease may therefore significantly impair absorption. However, there are usually sufficient hepatic stores of folate to last for five or six months if folate intake ceased (Table 2.8).

Vitamin B12 is found exclusively in food of animal origin (Table 2.7). On reaching the stomach, B12 is cleaved from food proteins by HCl and then bound to proteins similar to those that are responsible for its binding in the plasma – known as haptocorrins

(and previously termed 'R-binders'). Thus bound, B12 passes to the duodenum, where it is cleaved from the haptocorrin and binds to the glycoprotein Intrinsic Factor (IF). IF is essential for B12 absorption. It is highly resistant to enzymatic digestion and is able to transport B12 to the ileum, where the B12/IF complex binds its receptor, cubilin, and is endocytosed. Once passed into the circulation, B12 is bound to the transport protein transcobalamin.

From the outline above it is evident that vitamin B12 deficiency might arise from several mechanisms. First, vegan diets are likely to be lacking in B12. Any condition that results in achlorhydria (e.g. partial gastrectomy) will limit the cleavage of B12 from food-associated peptides and will also limit B12's availability for absorption. Disease in the terminal ileum may prevent the ability of the B12/IF complex to be taken up into enterocytes, while

Table 2.8 Causes of folate deficiency.

Inadequate dietary intake

Malabsorption
Coeliac disease, jejunal resection, tropical sprue

Increased requirement
Pregnancy, premature infants, chronic haemolytic anaemias, myelofibrosis, various malignant diseases

Increased loss
Long-term dialysis, congestive heart failure, acute liver disease

Complex mechanism
Anticonvulsant therapy,* ethanol abuse*

Note: * Only some cases with macrocytosis are folate deficient.

Table 2.9 **Mechanisms and causes of vitamin B12 deficiency.**

Inadequate intake
Veganism

Inadequate secretion of intrinsic factor
Pernicious anaemia
Total or partial gastrectomy
Congenital intrinsic factor deficiency (rare)

Inadequate release of B12 from food
Partial gastrectomy, vagotomy, gastritis, acid-suppressing drugs, alcohol abuse

Diversion of dietary B12
Abnormal intestinal bacterial flora multiple jejunal diverticula, small intestinal strictures, stagnant intestinal loops

Diphyllobothrium latum

Malabsorption
Crohn's disease, ileal resection, chronic tropical sprue

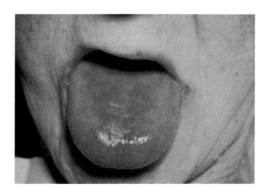

Figure 2.10 Glossitis in a woman with severe pernicious anaemia.

overgrowth of gut bacteria (or the presence of the fish tapeworm, *Diphyllobothrium latum*) can 'compete' for B12 in the gut and minimize the vitamin available for absorption.

However, perhaps the best known of the conditions leading to failure of B12 absorption is pernicious anaemia. This condition arises when auto-antibodies interfere with the production or function of intrinsic factor – with anti-parietal cell antibodies being associated with gastric atrophy and failure of IF secretion, or anti-intrinsic factors preventing the formation of the B12/IF complex or interfering with its ability to bind to cubilin. The causes of B12 deficiency are summarized in Table 2.9.

The clinical manifestations of B12 and folate deficiency

As well as the clinical effects of a macrocytic anaemia, with possible neutropenia and thrombocytopenia if severe, deficiencies of B12 and folate will occasionally produce a mild jaundice as destruction of poorly matured erythroid precursors releases the haem breakdown product bilirubin (see also Chapter 3 on haemolysis).

In addition, B12 deficiency is well known to produce a range of neurological symptoms, with a peripheral neuropathy (particularly affecting proprioception and vibration sense) being followed by demyelination of the dorsal and lateral columns of the spinal cord. This produces a pyramidal picture,

with increased tone, extensor plantars and sensory ataxia. This picture is termed subacute combined degeneration of the cord and its effects may be irreversible. The precise pathophysiology has not been established, but methionine is thought to have a role in the production and maintenance of myelin.

Additional tissues that may be affected include the gastrointestinal tract (from the mouth to the colon: Figure 2.10) and the skin.

Confirming a diagnosis of B12 or folate deficiency

Both B12 and folate deficiency will cause a macrocytic anaemia with megaloblastic erythropoiesis. The blood film will show oval macrocytes and hypersegmented neutrophils (again a consequence of delayed nuclear maturation – see Figure 2.11). The reticulocyte count is likely to be low for the degree of anaemia. A bone

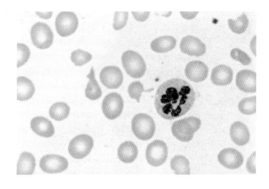

Figure 2.11 Blood film from a patient with pernicious anaemia showing oval macrocytes, other poikilocytes and a hypersegmented neutrophil.

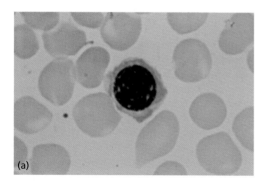

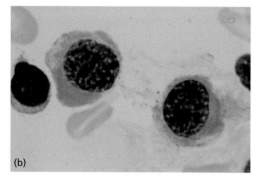

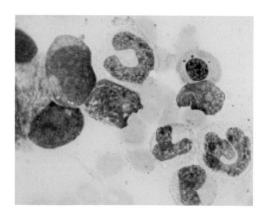

Figure 2.13 Two giant metamyelocytes near a normal-sized metamyelocyte in a marrow smear from a patient with untreated pernicious anaemia. There is also a megaloblast containing Howell–Jolly bodies (i.e. micronuclei).

Figure 2.12 (a) Early polychromatic normoblast from the marrow of a healthy subject. (b) Early polychromatic megaloblasts from a patient with severe pernicious anaemia. These cells are larger and have a more delicate, sieve-like nucleus containing smaller particles of condensed chromatin than the early polychromatic normoblast.

Testing for B12 deficiency may not be as straightforward as a simple serum vitamin B12 assay. The great majority of assayed B12 in the serum is protein bound as part of 'haptocorrin' – a form that is not functionally active; only B12 bound to the protein transcobalamin is physiologically available. Thus any condition that affects the distribution of B12-binding proteins in the serum can affect the result of B12 assays. Pregnancy and the oral contraceptive pill, for example, can give falsely low B12 results, while some myeloproliferative disorders (which increase haptocorrin

marrow aspirate, if performed, will show nuclear-cytoplasmic dyssynchrony and giant metamyelocytes (Figures 2.12, 2.13 and 2.14). The destruction of defective erythroid cells in the marrow will result in a mild increase in bilirubin and LDH levels (see also Chapter 3).

Folic acid levels may be assayed in the serum and in the red cells themselves. Serum folate tends to fluctuate rather more markedly in response to folate intake, so red cell folate levels are generally considered to be a better guide to functional folate status. However, the critical role of vitamin B12 in regenerating functional tetrahydrofolate means that low red cell folic acid levels may also be seen as a secondary effect in B12 deficiency. Moreover, although treating with folate supplementation when the primary defect is actually with B12 can temporarily ameliorate the haematological symptoms and signs, it will permit worsening of any B12-associated neurological pathology. B12 levels should therefore be routinely tested alongside folic acid levels.

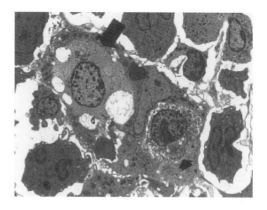

Figure 2.14 Electron micrograph of a bone marrow macrophage from a patient with severe pernicious anaemia. The cytoplasm of the macrophage contains two ingested megaloblasts (arrowed) at various stages of degradation.

production) give falsely high readings. If in doubt, the substrates of the cobalamin-requiring enzymes can be assayed: both homocysteine and methylmalonic acid levels will be high in true B12 deficiency.

Finding the cause of deficiency is also important. A clear dietary history, consideration of tests for malabsorption, endomyseal antibodies (if coeliac disease is suspected) and anti-intrinsic factor/antiparietal cell antibodies (to look for pernicious anaemia as a cause of B12 deficiency) should all be considered.

Treatment

In all cases, the underlying cause must be treated where possible. Folic acid supplementation orally is generally sufficient to treat folic acid deficiency, though care must be taken to ensure that coincident B12 deficiency is not missed. Oral B12 supplements may help where there is simple dietary deficiency of B12, but clearly in pernicious anaemia parenteral vitamin B12 administration by intramuscular injection is required.

Other causes of megaloblastosis

Conditions other than B12 and folate deficiency can cause megaloblastic erythropoiesis. Frequently, aberrations in the metabolism of B12 and folate are at the root of the megaloblastosis (consider the effects of methotrexate, which inhibits an enzyme critical for tetrahydrofolate production; or chronic nitrous oxide exposure, which can combine with the cobalt of cobalamin to inhibit its ability to function as an enzymatic cofactor); but any other drug or clinical condition that inhibits DNA synthesis will have a similar effect – as summarized in Table 2.10.

Normoblastic macrocytosis

Not all cases of macrocytic anaemia will be caused by megaloblastic changes in the marrow. Conditions in which macrocytosis is seen in the context of normoblastic erythropoiesis include alcohol excess (probably the commonest cause of macrocytosis in the UK), liver dysfunction and hypothyroidism. The mechanisms underlying the macrocytosis in these cases are not always fully defined. It is also possible for a marked expansion in erythroid output to produce a mild macrocytosis, since reticulocytes are slightly larger than more mature red cells. A summary of the causes of normoblastic macrocytosis is given in Table 2.11.

Spurious elevations in the mean cell volume may be seen in hyperglycaemia, thought to be a consequence of osmotic dysequilibrium between the red cells and the diluent used in preparing the cells for analysis.

Polycythaemia (erythrocytosis)

Just as perturbation of mechanisms controlling normal red cell production may result in anaemia, so dysregulation of these mechanisms may also result in too many red cells being produced. The term 'polycythaemia' refers to an excess of red cells, such that the packed cell volume (also known as the haematocrit) of peripheral blood is consistently elevated (>0.52 in adult males and >0.48 in adult females).

Table 2.10 Vitamin B12-independent and folate-independent causes of macrocytosis with megaloblastic haemopoiesis.

Abnormalities of nucleic acid synthesis

Drug therapy

    Antipurines (mercaptopurine, azathioprine)

    Antipyrimidines (fluorouracil, zidovudine (AZT))

    Others (hydroxycarbamide)

Orotic aciduria

Uncertain aetiology

Myelodysplastic syndromes,* erythroleukaemia

Some congenital dyserythropoietic anaemias

Note: *Some patients show normoblastic erythropoiesis.

Table 2.11 Causes of vitamin B12- and folate-independent macrocytosis with normoblastic erythropoiesis.

Normal neonates (physiological)

Chronic alcoholism*

Myelodysplastic syndromes*

Chronic liver disease*

Hypothyroidism

Normal pregnancy

Therapy with anticonvulsant drugs*

Haemolytic anaemia

Hypoplastic and aplastic anaemia

Myeloma

Note: *Some patients show B12- and folate-independent megaloblastic erythropoiesis.

Polycythaemia may result either from an increase in the total volume of red cells in the circulation (true polycythaemia) or from a decrease in the total plasma volume (apparent or relative polycythaemia). These are discussed in more detail in Chapter 11, but a brief overview of true polycythaemia is given below.

True polycythaemia

An absolute increase in circulating red cells may arise from dysregulation of any of the mechanisms controlling normal red cell production. Thus, hypoxia secondary to chronic pulmonary disease or cyanotic heart disease will increase erythropoietin production, with a resultant stimulation of erythroid drive in the bone marrow. High affinity haemoglobins, which fail to yield oxygen appropriately in the peripheral tissues, may also be responsible for an increased hypoxic signal and thus increased erythropoiesis. In normoxaemic conditions, inappropriate release of erythropoietin can occur in the context of renal tumours or polycystic kidney disease. Each of these cases will cause a true polycythaemia, but the ultimate cause in each case is extrinsic to the bone marrow: they are therefore termed 'secondary polycythaemias'.

Primary polycythaemia, also known as polycythaemia vera, arises from a defect in the haemopoietic system itself. It is characterized by the autonomous, epo-independent proliferation of erythroid precursors in the marrow. In the overwhelming majority of cases, this is due to the acquisition of a mutation in the gene for JAK2, a protein tyrosine kinase that is critical for the downstream signalling through the epo receptor. Over 95% of patients with polycythaemia vera have the JAK2 V617F mutation, which results in epo-independent red cell proliferation. A further mutation in exon 12 of the JAK2 gene has also been described, with similar effects.

The differential diagnosis of polycythaemia, and an approach to its management, are described in Chapter 11.

3

Haemolytic anaemias

Learning objectives

✓ To be able to define haemolysis and haemolytic anaemia

✓ To know the tests for recognizing:
  ✓ that red cells are being destroyed at an excessive rate, and
  ✓ that the marrow is producing cells at a rate in excess of normal

✓ To be able to classify haemolytic anaemias into congenital and acquired types, and to know the aetiological factors in each division

✓ To understand the difference between intravascular and extravascular haemolysis, and to recognise the laboratory features of each

✓ To understand the mode of inheritance, biochemical basis and clinical and laboratory features of hereditary spherocytosis (HS)

✓ To understand the normal role of glucose-6-phosphate dehydrogenase (G6PD) and the pathogenesis and clinical characteristics of the haemolytic syndromes associated with its deficiency

✓ To appreciate that disorders of globin function such as sickle cell disease are subtypes of haemolytic anaemia

✓ To understand the role of autoantibodies in the production of haemolytic anaemias and to know the types of disease with which they are associated

✓ To understand some causes of non-immune acquired haemolytic anaemias

Haemolysis describes the shortening of the lifespan of a mature red blood cell. Small or moderate reductions in red cell survival need not produce an obvious clinical effect: increased red cell output from the marrow, stimulated by erythropoietin, will be sufficient to compensate for the increased red cell destruction. However, more marked reductions in red cell lifespan – say to 5–10 days from the usual 120 days – will overwhelm the capacity of the marrow to expand erythroid output and will result in *haemolytic anaemia*.

This compensatory increase in erythroid output requires an adequately functioning bone marrow and effective erythropoiesis. However, a suboptimal marrow response is seen when there are insufficient haematinics, when the red cell precursors are damaged, when the marrow is infiltrated by malignant cells and when there is ineffective erythropoiesis, as in thalassaemia. In each of these conditions, haemolysis will result in anaemia more readily.

In the majority of haemolytic anaemias, the macrophages in the spleen, liver and bone marrow remove red cells from the circulation by phagocytosis. This is termed extravascular haemolysis. By contrast, in intravascular haemoysis, the red cells are caused to rupture and release their haemoglobin (Hb) directly into the circulation. The

Haematology Lecture Notes, Ninth edition. C.S.R. Hatton, N.C. Hughes-Jones, D. Hay and D. Keeling. © 2013 John Wiley & Sons, Ltd.
Published 2013 by John Wiley & Sons, Ltd.

intra/extravascular site of red cell destruction may give clues to the underlying aetiology of the haemolysis.

Laboratory evidence of haemolysis

Both biochemical and haematological laboratory investigations can provide evidence of haemolysis. When red cells are destroyed, either in the circulation or by the reticuloendothelial system, their haem group is converted first to biliverdin and then to bilirubin. Unconjugated bilirubin is insoluble and is transported to the liver bound to albumin; here it undergoes glucuronidation to facilitate its excretion. However, with increased red cell destruction the glucuronidase can become saturated, such that unconjugated bilirubin accumulates. Thus, haemolysis, whether intravascular or extravascular, will result in a rise in the unconjugated bilirubin concentration in the plasma.

Lactate dehydrogenase, an enzyme present in red cells, is also released from red cells as they are lysed. Breakdown of red cells intravascularly can result in very marked elevation of the serum LDH, while breaches in the red cell membrane caused by partial phagocytosis in extravascular haemolysis may also cause the serum LDH level to climb.

Specific biochemical markers of intravascular haemolysis include a reduction of serum haptoglobin. When red cells are lysed intravascularly, free haemoglobin is released; haptoglobin binds to this free haemoglobin, thereby limiting its potentially harmful oxidative effects. The haemoglobin–haptoglobin complex is scavenged by macrophages of the liver and spleen, resulting in a low or even absent plasma haptoglobin level. When the haptoglobin is saturated, free haem can bind to albumin to form methaemalbumin. This is also detectable biochemically. Unbound free haemoglobin can be detected in the plasma as well and may pass through the renal glomeruli to give free haemoglobin in the urine – haemoglobinuria (note the difference from haematuria, which describes the presence of intact red cells in the urine). Haemoglobin may also be taken up by the renal tubular cells and converted to the storage complex haemosiderin. This can be detected with Perls' stain of spun deposits of urine, both in shed tubular cells and extracellularly.

Haematologically, haemolysis is characterized by evidence of increased erythroid drive, manifest through an increased reticulocyte count. The number of reticulocytes in the blood is expressed either as a percentage of the total number of red cells or as an absolute number per litre of blood; in normal adults, the percentage is in the range of 0.5–3.0% and the absolute count is $20-100 \times 10^9$/L. An increase in the absolute reticulocyte count is an indication of increased erythropoietic activity and, in general, the higher the count, the greater the rate of delivery of viable red cells to the circulation. The reticulocyte percentage may increase up to 50% or more when erythropoietic activity is intense, as in brisk haemolysis – though it should be noted that reticulocytosis is not a feature *specific* to haemolysis; it will be observed whenever there is increased erythroid drive, such as during the response to acute blood loss, or following the replacement of B12, folic acid or iron in a setting of anaemia secondary to haematinic deficiency.

The slightly larger size of reticulocytes relative to mature red cells will lead to a small increase in the mean cell volume. As haemolysis will also increase the marrow's demand for folic acid, macrocytosis may also develop secondary to folate deficiency if this increased demand is not met by adequate intake (see also Chapter 2).

Aside from polychromasia due to reticulocytosis, the peripheral blood film in haemolysis will vary according to the underlying cause – specific morphological features of different haemolytic anaemias are described in more detail in the following sections. However, generally extravascular haemolysis is associated with spherocytosis on the peripheral blood film, due to the partial phagocytosis of red cells by the spleen, while intravascular haemolysis is characterized by red cell fragmentation (schistocytes).

In cases where examination of the bone marrow is undertaken, there will be evidence of increased erythropoiesis. A semiquantitative assessment of the degree of erythroid hyperplasia can be obtained by determining the myeloid/erythroid (M/E) ratio in the bone marrow. This is defined as the ratio between the number of cells of the neutrophil series (including mature granulocytes) and the number of erythroblasts in bone marrow, with a normal ratio being approximately 3:1. Marrows showing erythroid hyperplasia are also hypercellular, due to the replacement of fat cells by erythroblasts (Figure 3.1). In chronic haemolysis, haemopoietic tissue may extend into marrow cavities that usually contain only fat, and extramedullary haemopoiesis may develop in the liver, and spleen.

Again, these haematological features are not specific to haemolysis. Erythroid hyperplasia will also be seen after haemorrhage, in megaloblastic and sideroblastic anaemias (where erythropoiesis is markedly ineffective, see p. 11), as well as in neoplastic conditions such as polycythaemia and erythroleukaemia.

The laboratory features of haemolysis are summarized in Table 3.1.

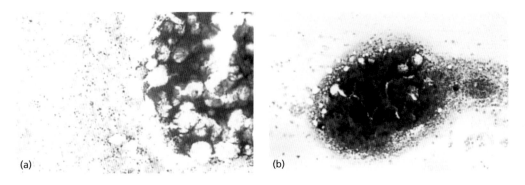

(a)   (b)

Figure 3.1 (a) A normocellular marrow fragment: about half its volume consists of haemopoietic cells (staining blue) and the remainder of unstained rounded fat cells. (b) A markedly hypercellular marrow fragment, as might be seen in the response to haemolysis: virtually all the fat cells are replaced by haemopoietic cells.

Clinical features of haemolysis

The haemolytic anaemias vary greatly in their clinical presentations. Some produce a mild, chronic, well-compensated haemolytic picture, while others manifest acutely with brisk haemolysis and a rapid drop in haemoglobin. The different clinical presentations seen with different causes of haemolysis are discussed further in the following sections, but common features include pallor, and jaundice secondary to the elevated bilirubin levels. Splenomegaly may be seen: in chronic haemolysis this may reflect the spleen's role in extramedullary erythropoiesis when the capacity of the normal marrow cavities to support red cell production is exceeded, while in florid acute haemolytic anaemias it may reflect the volume of red cells being phagocytosed in the spleen. Long-term complications of chronic haemolysis may include expansion of erythropoiesis in the marrow cavities, thinning of cortical bone, bone deformities (e.g. frontal and parietal bossing) and, very occasionally, pathological fractures. Pigment gallstones are seen commonly.

Patients with haemolytic conditions are also at risk of episodes of pure red cell aplasia. In this condition, which is typically the result of infection with parvovirus B19, there is a complete or near complete failure of erythroid maturation. Parvovirus binds to the carbohydrate P-antigen on erythroid progenitor cell surfaces and exerts a directly cytotoxic effect. In patients with a normal red cell lifespan, the temporary cessation of erythroid maturation it causes may produce a dip in the haemoglobin level, but it is usually clinically insignificant from a haematological perspective. However, in haemolytic states, the combination of reticulocytopenia and a pre-existing shortened red cell lifespan may have a catastrophic effect on the Hb level. Affected patients may require urgent red cell transfusion.

Table 3.1 **Laboratory findings indicative of haemoysis.**

Extravascular haemolysis	Intravascular haemolysis
Hyperbilirubinaemia (unconjugated)	Hyperbilirubinaemia (unconjugated)
	Reduced or absent serum haptoglobin
	Haemoglobinaemia, haemoglobinuria, haemosiderinuria
	Methaemalbuminaemia*
Increased serum lactate dehydrogenase (LDH)	Markedly increased serum LDH
Reticulocytosis	Reticulocytosis
Spherocytes	Red cell fragments (schistocytes)

Note: * Now rarely used in investigating a patient.

Classifying haemolytic anaemias and establishing a diagnosis

The laboratory and clinical features above describe general aspects of haemolytic states, but are not able to define the underlying cause of haemolysis. Many conditions are associated with a reduction in red cell survival, but these may be classified simply as either congenital or acquired. With the congenital causes, the underlying defect is typically intrinsic to the red cell itself, affecting the red cell membrane, its enzymes or its haemoglobin. Acquired causes, by contrast, are typically (but not exclusively) due to defects outside the red cell, and can be divided into those with an immune basis and those without. This overview is summarized in Figure 3.2 and the individual conditions are outlined below.

Congenital haemolytic anaemias

Haemolysis due to defects of the red cell membrane

Since the diameter of a normal red cell is similar to that of the smallest capillary lumen, it is essential for the red cell to be able to undergo significant deformations while traversing the circulation, while at the same time maintaining its structural integrity and avoiding

fragmentation. These contrasting requirements are accomplished through a flexible red cell cytoskeleton, which interacts with red cell phospholipid membrane. Key components of the cytoskeleton include α and β spectrin, actin and protein 4.1, while connections linking the cytoskeleton to the overlying red cell phospholipid bilayer include band 3, Rh-associated glycoprotein and glycophorin C (see Figure 3.3). Defects in any of these proteins can jeopardize the integrity of the red cell and shorten its lifespan.

Hereditary spherocytosis (HS)

The most common haemolytic anaemia due to a membrane defect is hereditary spherocytosis (HS), with 1 in 3000 people of Northern European ancestry being affected. About 60% of patients have mutations affecting the ankyrin gene, a critical linker between the phospholipid bilayer and the filamentous spectrin heterodimers of the red cell cytoskeleton. Loss of ankyrin then leads to secondary reductions in spectrin and protein 4.1. However, defects in other membrane-associated proteins may have similar effects, and the molecular nature of HS is consequently very heterogeneous. Defects in spectrin itself, band 3, protein 4.2 and the Rh complex have also been described, with a variety of different mutations defined. In a minority of cases no molecular cause can be identified. Although the bulk of kindreds show autosomal dominant inheritance, autosomal recessive patterns have also been identified in some families.

The consequence of uncoupling the connections between the membrane and the cytoskeleton is a tendency to release bilayer lipids in the form

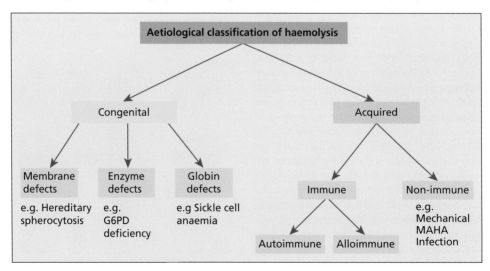

Figure 3.2 A classification of haemolytic anaemia by aetiology. Abbreviations: G6PD, glucose-6-phosphate dehydrogenase; MAHA, microangiopathic haemolytic anaemia.

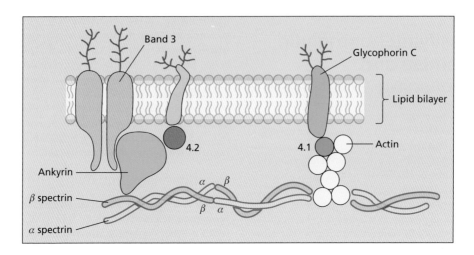

Figure 3.3 Schematic diagram of the red cell membrane cytoskeleton.

of cytoskeleton-free vesicles. This leads to a loss of membrane surface area, with cells adopting a spheroid rather than biconcave shape. Repeated passage through the spleen aggravates this spherocytic change. Being less deformable than normal red cells, the passage of spherocytes through the splenic cords is hampered: the trapped cells are engulfed and destroyed by splenic macrophages, leading to a reduction in red cell survival by extravascular haemolysis.

As might be expected from a condition so heterogeneous at the molecular level, HS is highly variable in its clinical presentation. Around 20% of all HS patients have mild disease with well-compensated haemolysis. These patients will have a near normal haemoglobin maintained by a higher than normal reticulocyte count, and will have only mild spherocytosis and mild splenomegaly. Indeed, such patients may not even present to medical attention until they develop complications of chronic haemolysis in adulthood (e.g. gallstones). The majority of patients have moderate disease characterized by a Hb concentration of 8–11g/dl, while a small percentage have severe disease requiring intermittent or even regular transfusions.

Complications of the chronic haemolysis in HS include the development of pigment gallstones (and possibly associated biliary obstruction). Aplastic crises may occur secondary to parvovirus B19 infection, and it should be noted than many otherwise trivial intercurrent infections can lead to episodes of increased haemolysis, sometimes requiring transfusion. Megaloblastic anaemia due to folate deficiency is also occasionally found, as in other chronic haemolytic disorders. This results from an increased requirement for folate by the hyperactive bone marrow, and is especially found when the diet is inadequate.

Diagnosis and management

The cardinal clinical features are a family history, mild jaundice, pallor and splenomegaly; but clearly these will not distinguish between HS and other forms of inherited haemolytic anaemia. Laboratory findings include the general features of haemolysis (anaemia, reticulocytosis and elevated plasma bilirubin, as above), but also the presence of spherocytes on the peripheral blood film (Figure 3.4). While spherocytes are also typically seen in patients with autoimmune haemolytic anaemia (see below), their presence in the context of a positive family history and a negative direct antiglobulin test will strongly suggest HS – and, indeed, no further diagnostic testing would be required in such patients.

Where more definitive evidence for the diagnosis is needed, the eosin-5-maleamide (EMA) binding test

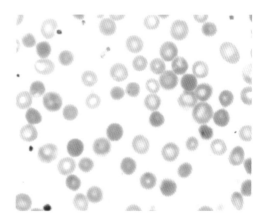

Figure 3.4 A blood film from a patient with HS showing many spherocytes.

may be used. EMA is a fluorescent dye that binds the transmembrane protein band 3 on the red cell surface. The extent of binding can be gauged by a flow cytometric analysis of a fluorescent signal from the cell surface (see Chapter 5 for further discussion of flow cytometry). HS, and other membrane disorders that result in disruption of the red cell cytoskeleton and its linkage to the phospholipid bilayer, will result in decreased EMA binding and a reduced fluorescent signal. An appreciation of which protein is affected may not be required for the clinical care of the patient; but if it is, or if other tests have yielded borderline results, the red cell membrane proteins may also be subject to electrophoresis on a denaturing polyacrylamide gel.

The treatment of HS should be tailored to the severity of the individual case. All patients should receive folic acid supplementation, in the light of their increased rate of erythropoiesis. Children with severe disease are likely to require splenectomy; this should also be considered for those with moderately severe disease. As well as markedly reducing haemolysis and lengthening the red cell lifespan, this will reduce the likelihood of developing long-term complications. Splenectomy will, however, increase the risk of significant infection, particularly from encapsulated organisms. This risk is especially marked in children under the age of 5, and splenectomy is therefore typically delayed until age 5–10 years. Preoperative preparation should include the administration of pneumococcal and meningococcal vaccine and *Haemophilus influenzae* type b vaccine, and prophylactic penicillin V is advised lifelong post splenectomy, in an attempt to prevent the development of serious infection from *Neisseria meningitidis*, *Streptococcus pneumoniae* and other encapsulated organisms.

Hereditary elliptocytosis and hereditary pyropoikilocytosis

Hereditary eliptocytosis (HE) is also a relatively common condition, especially in regions where malaria is endemic. As with HS, it is heterogeneous at both a molecular and clinical level. The majority of kindreds have defects in α spectrin, though other components of the red cell cytoskeleton may be affected. While most patients are clinically asymptomatic, some will have a chronic symptomatic haemolytic anaemia. All show the very characteristic red cell shape on peripheral blood films (Figure 3.5).

Where there is severe disturbance of the multimerization of spectrin, patients usually have a severe haemolytic anaemia from infancy, with bizarre peripheral blood morphology, including microspherocytes and poikilocytes. Such patients are

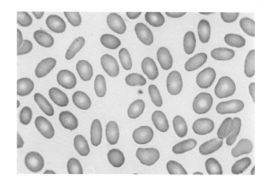

Figure 3.5 A blood film from a patient with hereditary elliptocytosis showing a high proportion of elliptical red cells.

described as having hereditary pyropoikilocytosis, although molecular analysis shows that this is in fact a homozygous or compound heterozygous state for the mutations that cause HE.

Haemolysis due to abnormalities of red cell enzymes

Haemolytic anaemias may also result from congenital abnormalities of the enzymes required for energy transfer in glucose metabolism. The red cell needs a continuous supply of energy for the maintenance of membrane flexibility and cell shape, the regulation of sodium and potassium pumps, and the maintenance of Hb in the reduced ferrous form. Since mature red cells lack mitochondria, there is a reliance principally on the anaerobic glycolytic pathway for glucose metabolism and ATP generation.

There is also an alternative direct oxidative pathway for glucose metabolism, the pentose-phosphate shunt, in which glucose-6-phosphate is directly oxidized, eventually leading to the production of metabolites that can rejoin the anaerobic glycolytic pathway. Although this shunt does not yield ATP directly, it is capable of reducing NADP+ to NADPH, which in turn can be oxidized to maintain reduced glutathione (GSH). The significance of the pentose-phosphate shunt is therefore its ability to provide a pool of 'reducing activity' that can be used to keep the sulphydryl groups of haemoglobin, red cell enzymes and membrane proteins in their functional reduced forms (see Figure 3.6).

Glucose-6-phosphate dehydrogenase deficiency

Deficiency of glucose-6-phosphate dehydrogenase (G6PD), the first enzyme of the pentose-phosphate

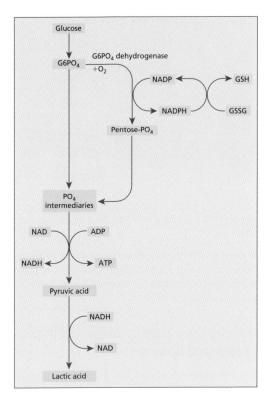

Figure 3.6 A schematic diagram of the pathway of glucose metabolism in the red cell, to show the important role of G6PD. A decreased activity of the enzyme leads to a deficiency of the reducing compounds NADPH and GSH.

shunt, will prevent the normal generation of NADPH, with subsequent erythrocyte sensitivity to oxidative stress. The molecular basis of G6PD deficiency is highly variable, with various point mutations in the G6PD gene on the X chromosome resulting in enzymes with altered activity, kinetics and interactions. The normal G6PD enzyme is designated type B and is the prevalent form worldwide; G6PD type A is a normal variant found in approximately 20% of healthy individuals of African ancestry. Defective forms of G6PD include the A– African variant in which the enzyme activity is reduced to approximately one tenth of its normal function, and the Mediterranean variant in which the enzyme activity is even more markedly limited, at 1–3% of normal. Together, these two mutations account for >95% of all cases of G6PD deficiency.

Since the gene for G6PD is found on the X chromosome, affected individuals are male (homozygous women are affected as well, but are unusual; skewed lionization may also give reduced enzyme activity in some heterozygous women). It has been estimated that as many as 400 million people worldwide are affected, with the prevalence being high in areas where malaria is endemic. It has been shown that the deficiency affords some protection against *plasmodium falciparum* malaria, with heterozygous females infected with malaria having lower parasite counts in their red cells than women without G6PD deficiency. Deficiency of the enzyme is found in about 20% of individuals of west and central African origin and is also found to a varying extent in southern Europe, the Middle East, India, Thailand and southern China. It is very rare in people of northern European origin.

Since G6PD has a critical role in maintaining the pool of reducing power in the erythrocyte, patients with low levels of the enzyme are poorly protected against oxidative challenge – with some medications and even foods resulting in marked oxidative damage to the red cell. When the red cell is exposed to oxidants, haemoglobin is converted to methaemoglobin and denatured. Denatured haemoglobin then precipitates forming inclusions in the red cell (termed Heinz bodies and detected by supravital staining, as in Figure 3.7). Heinz bodies, and the portion of the red cell membrane to which they become attached, are removed by splenic macrophages as the red cells pass through the spleen; the resulting inclusion-free cells display unstained areas at their periphery ('bite' cells, seen in Figure 3.8). Red cells with oxidative membrane damage will be removed extravascularly by the spleen, though acute responses to a severe oxidative challenge may also provoke intravascular haemolysis.

Oxidant drugs that may bring about this type of haemolytic anaemia include antimalarial drugs (e.g. primaquine and chloroquine), sulphonamides, nitrofurantoin, chloramphenicol, aspirin (in high doses), dapsone, phenacetin and vitamin K analogues.

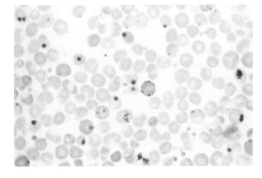

Figure 3.7 Membrane-bound Heinz bodies consisting of denatured haemoglobin (supravital staining with methyl violet).

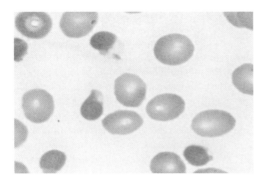

Figure 3.8 'Bite' cells in the blood film of a patient with G6PD deficiency who had received primaquine. These red cells are irregular in shape, are abnormally dense and show a poorly staining area just beneath part of the cell membrane (MGG stain).

A number of screening tests and assays for detecting G6PD deficiency are available. These are based on assessing the production of NADPH by red cells in the presence of an excess of glucose-6-phosphate. The NADPH is detected spectrophotometrically, by its ability to reduce nitroblue tetrazolium (NBT) in the presence of an electron transfer agent, or by its ability to fluoresce in ultraviolet light.

A variety of clinical syndromes may be associated with G6PD variants that have reduced enzyme activity. The commonest of these is episodic acute haemolysis. For most of the time, patients with the two common G6PD variants (A– and Mediterranean types) are well and have normal Hb concentrations with only a slight shortening of the red cell lifespan. Episodes of haemolytic anaemia develop during infections or following exposure to oxidant drugs and chemicals. Haemolysis typically begins 1–3 days following exposure to the oxidative stressor, with anaemia being maximal about 7–10 days after exposure. The extent of the fall in Hb concentration is partly dependent on the amount and nature of the drug being given, and partly on the extent of the reduction of enzyme activity. During this time, the patient may report dark urine due to haemoglobinuria. A subtype of acute haemolysis is favism, a syndrome in which an acute haemolytic anaemia occurs after the ingestion of the broad bean (*Vicia fava*) in individuals with a deficiency of G6PD (commonly of the Mediterranean type). Favism usually affects children; severe anaemia develops rapidly and is often accompanied by haemoglobinuria. Fava beans contain two β-glycosides, vicine and convicine, which generate free radicals and consequently oxidize GSH and other red cell constituents.

Although the majority of patients with G6PD deficiency have episodic haemolytic episodes, some patients with severe enzyme defects have a more chronic haemolytic picture, with oxidative exacerbations. In these patients, the chronic haemolysis is principally extravascular.

A further possible presentation of G6PD deficiency is in infancy, with hyperbilirubinaemia. A combination of oxidative damage to red cells alongside immaturity of the bilirubin-conjugating system can lead to hyperbilirubinaemia, sometimes necessitating exchange transfusion. Affected individuals recover completely after the neonatal period, but may develop episodic acute haemolysis during later life.

Treatment of G6PD deficiency

Treatment generally focuses on the avoidance of oxidative precipitants to haemolysis. In many cases, haemolysis is self limiting: in patients with the A– variant, for example, after about 10 days the Hb concentration starts to climb and may reach normal levels, even with continuation of the offending oxidant drug. This is because in these patients only the older red cells have sufficiently low G6PD levels to be affected. As the reticulocyte count rises, so the effect of exposure to the oxidant is diminished. For patients with the Mediterranean variant, in whom the average enzyme activity is lower haemolytic episodes may not be self-limiting, and packed red cell transfusion may be required in cases of severe haemolysis.

Other red cell enzyme deficiencies causing haemolysis

G6PD is not the only enzyme deficiency that can result in haemolysis. Pyruvate kinase deficiency is another relatively common example, affecting individuals of all ethnic origins. As with G6PD deficiency, it is thought to have a protective role in *plasmodium falciparum* infection, explaining its relatively high prevalence. At a molecular level it is a highly heterogeneous condition, with most affected patients being compound heterozygotes. This heterogeneity is reflected in the clinical presentation, but there is usually a chronic haemolytic anaemia and some patients may benefit from splenectomy.

Haemolysis due to haemoglobin defects

The third category of congenital haemolytic anaemias relates to defects in the structure of haemoglobin. These conditions are summarized as part of the classification of haemolytic anaemias, but are discussed in more detail in Chapter 4. Briefly, structural variants of the globin chains may affect the lifespan of the red cell, with sickle cell anaemia being the best-described example. A tendency of the HbS variant to polymerize under conditions of low oxygen tension leads to distortion of the erythrocyte into the well-recognized sickle shape. The distorted cells are subject to both intra- and extravascular haemolysis.

Acquired haemolytic anaemias

In the acquired haemolytic anaemias, red cells may be destroyed either by immunological or by non-immunological mechanisms.

Immune haemolytic anaemias

In these conditions, antigens on the surface of red cells react with antibodies sometimes with complement activation. IgG-coated red cells interact with the Fc receptors on macrophages in the spleen, and are then either completely or partially phagocytosed. When the phagocytosis is partial, the damaged cell will return to the circulation as a spherocyte. Red cells that are also coated with the activated complement component C3 may interact with C3 receptors on macrophages and are usually completely phagocytosed. In most instances where complement is activated, the cascade sequence only proceeds as far as C3 deposition on the cell surface. In a few instances, activation of complement proceeds further and permits deposition of the membrane attack complex (C5–C9) with resultant intravascular haemolysis.

The immune haemolytic anaemias may be due to autoantibodies; that is, antibodies formed against one or more antigenic constituents of the individual's own tissues. These include autoimmune haemolytic anaemia (AIHA) and some drug-related haemolytic anaemias. However, it is also possible to develop alloimmune haemolytic anaemia, consequent on the production of antibodies against red cells from another individual, as in haemolytic transfusion reactions and haemolytic disease of the newborn (Chapter 15). A further mechanism by which immune dysregulation can result in haemolysis is found in the rare condition paroxysmal nocturnal haemoglobinuria (PNH), which arises when an acquired defect in the red cell membrane leads to complement-mediated haemolysis (see Box 3.1). Each of these subtypes of immune haemolysis is discussed in further detail below.

Autoimmune haemolytic anaemias

A classification of the autoimmune haemolytic anaemias is given in Table 3.2. The temperature dependence of the autoantibody's binding affinity for its red cell surface antigen will determine the clinical picture. 'Warm' autoantibodies react best with the red cell antigen at 37°C and are usually of IgG subtype. 'Cold' antibodies react best at temperatures below 32°C (usually below 15°C) and, since they are usually of IgM subtype, are capable of agglutinating red cells.

Warm AIHA

In idiopathic warm AIHA, haemolysis dominates the clinical picture and no evidence can be found of any other disease. In secondary AIHA, the haemolysis is associated with a primary disease such as chronic lymphocytic leukaemia or systemic lupus erythematosus (SLE). Some 50–70% of 'warm' autoantibodies show specificity for the Rh antigen system (see Chapter 15) and some of the remainder for other blood group antigen systems. The pathological mechanism by which these antibodies arise is unclear.

The antibody-coated red cells undergo partial or complete phagocytosis in the spleen and by the Kupffer cells of the liver. There may be partial activation of the complement cascade in addition, although completion to the membrane attack complex of complement is rare – a likely consequence of the activity of the complement regulatory proteins, factors I and H.

The clinical presentation of warm AIHA is highly variable but, unlike cold AIHA, it is unrelated to ambient temperature. Patients are usually over the age of 50. Some patients with florid haemolysis are very ill with an acute onset of severe anaemia; others have

Table 3.2 Classification of AIHAs.

Caused by warm-reactive antibodies

Idiopathic

Secondary (chronic lymphocytic leukaemia, lymphoma, systemic lupus erythematosus (SLE), some drugs)

Caused by cold-reactive antibodies

Cold haemagglutinin disease

Idiopathic

Secondary (*Mycoplasma pneumoniae* infection, infectious mononucleosis, lymphomas)

Paroxysmal cold haemoglobinuria

Idiopathic

Secondary (some viral infections, congenital and tertiary syphilis)

few or no symptoms and a mild chronic anaemia or even a compensated haemolytic state. Mild jaundice is common and splenomegaly may be found.

Haematological findings include anaemia, spherocytosis (Figure 3.9), reticulocytosis, occasional nucleated red cells in the peripheral blood and sometimes a neutrophil leucocytosis. However, the critical diagnostic investigation is the direct antiglobulin test (also known as the direct Coombs' test). In this test, washed red cells from the patient are incubated with an antihuman globulin, which is able to bind to antibodies on the red cell surface. Being divalent, the antihuman globulin can bind IgG from two red cells, and is thus able to agglutinate cells that are coated with antibody. Such agglutination of red cells constitutes a positive direct antiglobulin test. Cells that are not coated with IgG will remain unagglutinated. The test can also be made specific for individual subtypes of IgG and for complement components that may be found on the red cell surface in AIHA. It should be noted, however, that a positive direct antiglobulin test does not always imply active haemolysis: studies of healthy blood donors suggest that up to 1 in 10,000 of the population will have a positive test without haematological consequences.

In most patients, the haemolysis can be limited by treatment with prednisolone, which is initially given in high doses. If there is no response to steroids, or if the reduction in haemolysis is not maintained when the dose of steroids is lowered, splenectomy or alternative immunosuppressive therapy should be considered. The anti-CD20 monoclonal antibody rituximab, as well as immunosuppressants such as azathioprine or cyclophosphamide, may be beneficial in reducing autoantibody production. In patients with severe anaemia and circulatory compromise, the least incompatible ABO- and Rh-matched blood should be transfused. However, transfusion is avoided wherever possible in AIHA, as even transfused cells may become coated with antibody and will have a relatively short half-life.

Cold haemagglutinin disease (CHAD)

Since cold antibodies react with red cells only at temperatures below about 32°C, they typically bind to the red cell surface in the cooler superficial blood vessels of the peripheries. Here, the presence of the antibody permits complement fixation. Red cells bearing complement will be susceptible to partial or complete phagocytosis in the spleen, but completion of the complement cascade may also be seen, with the insertion of the membrane attack complex and consequent intravascular haemolysis. Since the cold antibodies are typically of the IgM subtype, their pentameric structure permits direct agglutination of red cells coated with antibody; they are therefore sometimes termed cold agglutinins. This is readily seen in blood films made at room temperature (Figure 3.10).

Symptoms due to cold AIHA are worse during cold weather. Exposure to cold provokes acrocyanosis (coldness, purplish discolouration and numbness of fingers, toes, ear lobes and the nose), due to the formation of agglutinates of red cells in the vessels of the skin. The direct activation of the complement system leads to red cell lysis and, consequently, to haemoglobinaemia and haemoglobinuria.

A direct antiglobulin test will reveal that complement proteins are bound to the red cell surface, though the cold antibody itself frequently dissociates from the red cells during the washing phase of the test and may not be detected. The cold agglutinin in chronic idiopathic CHAD is usually a monoclonal IgM antibody, normally with anti-I specificity (I and i are the names given to carbohydrate antigens on the surface of red cells; adult red cells contain more

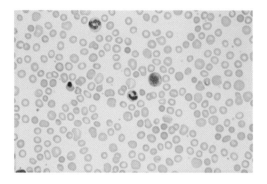

Figure 3.9 Blood film from a patient with idiopathic AIHA (warm-reactive antibody) showing prominent spherocytosis and polychromasia.

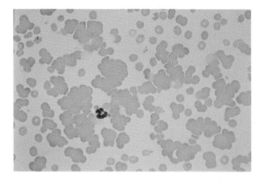

Figure 3.10 Numerous red cell agglutinates on a blood film from a patient with idiopathic CHAD.

I than i determinants). The anti-I titre at 4°C may be as high as 1:2000 to 1:500,000 (normal, 1:10–40). It should also be noted that a monoclonal cold agglutinin may also be seen with several B cell lymphomas.

Rarely, patients with Mycoplasma pneumonia or infectious mononucleosis may develop acute self-limiting cold agglutinin-induced haemolytic anaemia, due to the production of polyclonal IgM antibodies with anti-I or anti-i specificity, respectively.

Chronic idiopathic CHAD is managed initially simply by keeping the patient warm. However, some patients remain symptomatic and treatment is required. Unlike warm AIHA, glucocorticoids and splenectomy tend to be of limited use. Treatment with rituximab may be effective.

Other causes of haemolytic anaemia with an immune element to their pathogenesis include paroxysmal nocturnal haemoglobinuria, paroxysmal cold haemoglobinuria and some drug-related haemolytic anaemias (see Box 3.1).

Box 3.1

Paroxysmal nocturnal haemoglobinuria (PNH)

This rare, clonal disorder arises as a consequence of somatic mutation of the *PIG-A* gene in a multipotent haemopoietic stem cell. The product of the *PIG-A* gene is critical for forming the glycosyl-phosphatidylinositol (GPI) anchor, which links many membrane proteins to the phospholipid bilayer. Among the many GPI-anchored proteins are CD55 and CD59, also known as decay-accelerating factor and the membrane inhibitor of reactive lysis. These proteins are critical regulators of the complement pathway. Consequently, cells that lack the GPI anchor have reduced or absent CD55 and CD59 on their cell membranes, and are extremely sensitive to complement-mediated intravascular haemolysis.

The haemolysis of PNH is generally chronic, although there may be acute exacerbations. Thrombosis is another clinical feature of PNH; while the mechanisms underlying it are not fully understood, it is known that some components of the fibrinolytic pathway are GPI linked, and free haemoglobin released in intravascular haemolysis may also have an activating effect on vascular endothelial cells.

The diagnosis is usually based on flow cytometry for key GPI-anchored proteins CD55 and CD59. Newer techniques to diagnose PNH include FLAER (fluorescent labelled aerolysin), in which a bacterially derived aeolysin binds to the GPI anchor itself; thus the absence of fluorescence due to FLAER in a population of myeloid cells will indicate the presence of a PNH clone. Treatment may be supportive (folic

---

acid and iron supplementation, anticoagulation where needed), although newer treatments targeting the underlying pathophysiology include Eculizumab, a monoclonal antibody against the C5 component of complement.

Paroxysmal cold haemoglobinuria

This rare disease is caused by an IgG antibody with anti-P specificity (P is a glycolipid red cell antigen). The antibody, called the Donath–Landsteiner antibody, is capable of binding complement and has a particular thermal profile of activity. The antibody and early complement components bind to red cells at 4°C but lysis occurs only on warming to 37°C. A rapid screening test therefore consists of incubating the patient's red cells and serum at 4°C and then warming the mixture to 37°C (the Donath–Landsteiner test). As might be predicted, patients suffer from acute episodes of marked haemoglobinuria due to severe intravascular haemolysis when exposed to the cold. An acute transient form associated with a viral infection (e.g. influenza, mumps, Epstein–Barr virus) affects children. The chronic form is usually seen in adults and is associated with syphilis. Idiopathic chronic PCH is rare.

Drug-induced haemolytic anaemia

There are several mechanisms by which drugs can induce a haemolytic anaemia. In some cases, the drug may act as a hapten and bind to red cell membrane proteins, inducing antibody formation. Penicillins, especially in high doses, have been implicated in this form of haemolytic anaemia. Alpha methyldopa is another drug well known to produce haemolytic anaemia in some patients, through the interaction of autoantibodies with the red cell surface, even in the absence of the drug – a mechanism clearly distinct from the hapten mechanism or immune complex effect. Treatment in each case focuses on the withdrawal of the offending drug; as with other causes of immune haemolysis, transfusion is avoided where possible.

Non-immune haemolytic anaemias

Mechanical damage to red cells

Several of the mechanical causes of acquired non-immune haemolytic anaemia are summarized in Table 3.3. Red cells are mechanically damaged when

Table 3.3 Causes of acquired non-immune haemolytic anaemias.

Mechanical trauma to red cells

Abnormalities in the heart and large blood vessels

Aortic valve prostheses (Figure 3.11), severe aortic valve disease

Microangiopathic haemolytic anaemia

Haemolytic uraemic syndrome, thrombotic thrombocytopenic purpura, metastatic malignancy, malignant hypertension, disseminated intravascular coagulation

March haemoglobinuria

Burns

Infections

Clostridium perfringens (welchii), malaria (Figures 3.12 and 3.13), bartonellosis

Drugs,* chemicals and venoms

Oxidant drugs and chemicals, arsine, acute lead poisoning, copper toxicity, venoms of certain spiders and snakes

Hypersplenism

Note: * Some drugs cause haemolysis by immune mechanisms.

they impact upon abnormal surfaces. These may include cardiac valve prostheses in valve-associated haemolysis, or activated vascular endothelium in the microangiopathic haemolytic anaemias. In disseminated intravascular coagulation (see Chapter 14) inappropriate activation of the coagulation cascade produces fibrin strands which are thought to cause mechanical destruction of red cells. Such damage usually results in the presence of red cell fragments in the blood film and, since the red cells are damaged

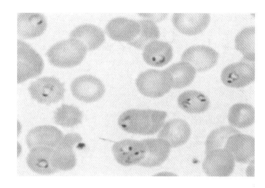

Figure 3.12 Blood film from a patient with *Plasmodium falciparum* malaria showing several parasitized red cells. Red cells heavily parasitized with malaria may be subject to intravascular lysis.

intravascularly, there may also be haemoglobinaemia, haemoglobinuria and an undetectable plasma haptoglobin.

Non-immune haemolytic anaemia due to drugs

While immune mechanisms of drug-induced haemolysis are well described, there are also non-immune mechanisms by which the red cell lifespan may be shortened. Chemicals, such as benzene, toluene and saponin, which are fat solvents, act on the red cell membrane directly and disrupt its lipid components, inducing haemolysis. In addition, certain drugs, such as primaquine, the sulphonamides and phenacetin, which oxidize and denature Hb and other cell components in people with a deficiency of G6PD, can, if

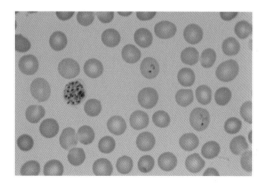

Figure 3.13 Blood film from a patient with *Plasmodium vivax* malaria showing two parasitized red cells, each containing a single parasite (ring form or early trophozoite and an ameboid late trophozoite). Another red cell contains a schizont. Some of the parasitized cells are slightly enlarged.

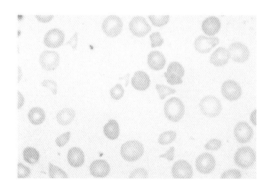

Figure 3.11 Fragmented red cells (schistocytes) in the blood film of a patient with a malfunctioning aortic valve prosthesis.

given in a large enough dose, also affect normal red cells. When given in conventional doses, the two oxidant drugs dapsone and sulphasalazine will also cause haemolysis in most patients.

Hypersplenism

Hypersplenism describes the reduction in the lifespan of red cells, granulocytes and platelets that may be found in patients with splenomegaly due to any cause. The cytopenias found in patients with enlarged spleens are also partly caused by increased pooling of blood cells within the spleen and an increased plasma volume; the magnitude of both these effects is proportioned to spleen size. In some haematological diseases in which anaemia is caused by a congenital or acquired defect of the red cell or impaired red cell formation, hypersplenism may have a role in worsening the anaemia, and splenectomy may be needed to address the effect.

Disorders of globin synthesis

Learning objectives

✓ To understand the normal structure and function of haemoglobin

✓ To understand how the globin components of haemoglobin change during development, and postnatally

✓ To understand the mechanisms by which the thalassaemias arise

✓ To appreciate the clinical presentations and complications of thalassaemia

✓ To appreciate the contribution of haemolysis and ineffective erythropoiesis to the pathophysiology of thalassaemia

✓ To understand the pathophysiology of sickle cell anaemia

✓ To be able to describe the clinical presentation and complications of sickle cell anaemia

✓ To understand the role of haemoglobin electrophoresis and high performance liquid chromatography in the investigation of globin disorders

✓ To appreciate the many other haemoglobin variants associated with disease

Normal structure and function of haemoglobin

Haemoglobin is critical to the normal function of the red cell, the fundamental role of which is the transport of oxygen from the lungs to the tissues. The normal haemoglobin molecule comprises two 'alpha-like' globin polypeptide chains and two 'beta-like' globin chains; each globin molecule is associated with a haem group, which comprises a porphyrin ring with iron in its ferrous form at the centre. It is to the iron in this haem group that oxygen binds.

In shifting between the oxygen-unbound and bound states, the haemoglobin molecule undergoes conformational change, which enhances its affinity for the binding of subsequent molecules of oxygen. The physiological consequence of this is haemoglobin's sigmoidal oxygen binding curve, which enables it to load oxygen effectively in situations of high oxygen tension, yet also to release it effectively in the low oxygen tension of the peripheral tissues.

In addition, several other ligands can allosterically influence the binding of oxygen to the haem groups. 2,3-diphosphoglycerate (2,3-DPG), a by-product of glucose metabolism in the cell, can bind to the β globin chains and allosterically decrease the affinity of haemoglobin for oxygen, thus shifting the oxygen dissociation curve to the right and encouraging the release of oxygen to the tissues. A fall in the pH in the peripheral tissues or an increase in the CO_2 concentration (the Bohr effect)

Haematology Lecture Notes, Ninth edition. C.S.R. Hatton, N.C. Hughes-Jones, D. Hay and D. Keeling. © 2013 John Wiley & Sons, Ltd.
Published 2013 by John Wiley & Sons, Ltd.

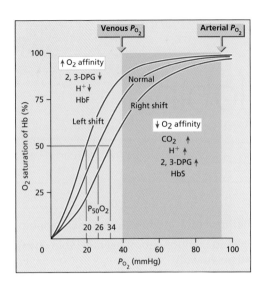

Figure 4.1 Oxygen dissociation curves of human blood.

both have similar consequences, such that the release of oxygen from the haemoglobin molecule to the tissues can be enhanced in the setting of increased metabolic demand (Figure 4.1).

The globin chain composition of haemoglobin can also influence its oxygen affinity. Although all normal haemoglobins consist of two pairs of distinct globin polypeptides, the precise nature of these globin chains changes during intrauterine and postnatal life. The α chains are encoded on chromosome 16 and are arranged in the order in which they are expressed during development: the embryonic ζ globin chain first, followed by the adult α globin chain. The β-like globins are encoded on chromosome 11 and again are found in the order of their expression: the

embryonic ε chain, followed by the fetal γ globin and the adult β globin. Thus, the complete haemoglobin molecule varies in its composition during development: Hb Gower ($\zeta_2\varepsilon_2$ and $\alpha_2\varepsilon_2$) and Hb Portland ($\zeta_2\gamma_2$) are the earliest forms seen, followed by the predominant fetal haemoglobin HbF ($\alpha_2\gamma_2$), which persists for several months postnatally, but contributes barely any of the normal adult complement of haemoglobins. The major adult haemoglobin is HbA ($\alpha_2\beta_2$), with a much smaller contribution from HbA2 ($\alpha_2\delta_2$ – usually 1.5–3.5% of adult haemoglobins). The fetal haemoglobin HbF has a higher oxygen affinity than the adult haemoglobins, facilitating transfer of oxygen from the maternal to the fetal circulation.

Normally, the synthesis of α-like and β-like chains is balanced, although the mechanisms permitting this balance remain incompletely understood. An imbalance between the production of α and β chains is the pathophysiological basis of the thalassaemias. Disorders of haemoglobin structure may also arise in the absence of imbalance between the α and β globin chains, with sickle cell anaemia being the principal example discussed in this chapter.

Thalassaemia

The thalassaemias are among the commonest genetic disorders in the world and are also among the most intensively studied from a molecular perspective. Notwithstanding this, their treatment is frequently only supportive and they are responsible for a huge burden of morbidity and mortality worldwide – most especially in countries that are economically least able to meet this challenge (Figure 4.2).

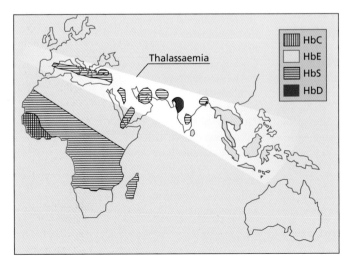

Figure 4.2 Distribution of the genes for the major Hb variants (S, E, C, D) and thalassemia.

The thalassaemias are divided into two main groups, the α-thalassaemias and the β-thalassaemias, depending on whether the defect lies in the synthesis of α- or β-globin chains respectively. The pathophysiology reflects the impact of an imbalance in the expression of α and β globin chains. The chains which are present in excess will precipitate in the precursor red cells, leading to their premature death prior to release from the bone marrow (ineffective erythropoiesis); in those cells that do mature sufficiently to reach the circulation, precipitated globin chains result in oxidative damage to the red cell membrane, with a consequent shortening of the red cell lifespan (haemolysis).

The resulting anaemia leads to an increased erythroid drive; as this manifests in further ineffective erythropoiesis, there is further expansion of the marrow into bones not typically used for haemopoiesis, and into the spleen. The long-term consequences of thalassaemia therefore include splenomegaly, bony deformities and iron excess (see Chapter 2 for details of the impact of chronic anaemia on iron absorption), as well as chronic anaemia.

The severity of the disease will vary greatly according to the degree of globin chain imbalance. The clinical phenotypes of patients with thalassaemia are discussed in more detail below.

α-Thalassaemia

α-thalassaemia is seen with the greatest frequency in south-east Asia (Thailand, the Malay Peninsula and Indonesia) and west Africa. The prevalence in these countries is in the region of 20–30%. It is also prevalent in southern Europe and the Middle East, but sporadic cases have been reported in most racial groups. Each chromosome 16 has an α-globin locus consisting of two α-globin genes plus the regulatory sequences essential for their normal expression. In most patients with α-thalassaemia, there is a deletion of one or more of the α-globin genes; there are occasional cases that are the consequence of non-deletional defects.

Deletion of one or two genes causes an asymptomatic condition with minor haematological features; deletion of three of the four α-globin genes causes a more severe imbalance of α:β-globin chains and results in haemoglobin H disease; and loss of all four α-globin genes causes Hb Bart's hydrops fetalis syndrome. Deletions may encompass both α genes on the same chromosome (termed α^0, as no α-globin will be transcribed from the affected chromosome) or may involve only a single α gene (called α^+, as the residual α gene on the affected chromosome may still be expressed) (Figure 4.3). Both the α^0-thalassaemia and the α^+-thalassaemia alleles are found in south-east

Asia and the Mediterranean region. The main type of α-thalassaemia found in west Africa, the Middle East, India and the Pacific Islands is α^+; α^0 is very rare here. As might be predicted, in populations in which the α^0-thalassaemia determinant is rare, HbH disease is also rare and Hb Bart's hydrops fetalis syndrome is not found. In northern Thailand, where both α^+- and α^0-thalassaemia traits are particularly common, 0.4% of deliveries are stillbirths due to Hb Bart's hydrops fetalis syndrome and HbH disease is found in about 1% of the population.

α^+-Thalassaemia trait (deletion of one α globin gene)

This is seen when an individual inherits the α^+-thalassaemia allele from one parent and a normal chromosome 16 from the other parent (i.e. heterozygotes for the α^+ determinant). Affected individuals are asymptomatic, although they have minor haematological changes such as slight reductions in mean cell volume (MCV) and mean cell haemoglobin (MCH).

α^0-Thalassaemia trait (deletion of both α-globin genes on one chromosome 16)

This is seen in heterozygotes for an α^0-thalassaemia allele. The Hb is either normal or slightly reduced and the MCV and MCH are low. (Similar haematological changes are seen in homozygotes for the α^+-thalassaemia determinant who also have a total of two α-globin genes deleted.)

Haemoglobin H disease (deletion of three α-globin genes)

This chronic haemolytic anaemia results from the inheritance of both the α^+- and α^0-thalassaemia alleles, leaving one functioning α-globin gene per cell. α-globin chains are produced at very low rates, leaving a considerable excess of β-chains, which combine to form tetramers (β_4). This tetramer is known as HbH. HbH is unstable and precipitates as the erythrocytes age, forming rigid membrane-bound inclusions that are removed during the passage of affected red cells through the spleen. The damage to the membrane brought about by this removal results in a shortened red cell lifespan.

The clinical picture of HbH disease is very variable. Most patients are moderately affected, with a mild anaemia of 7–11g/dl and markedly hypochromic, microcytic indices (Figure 4.4). Supravital staining of the blood film demonstrates cells with many HbH inclusions, giving a characteristic 'golf-ball' appearance.

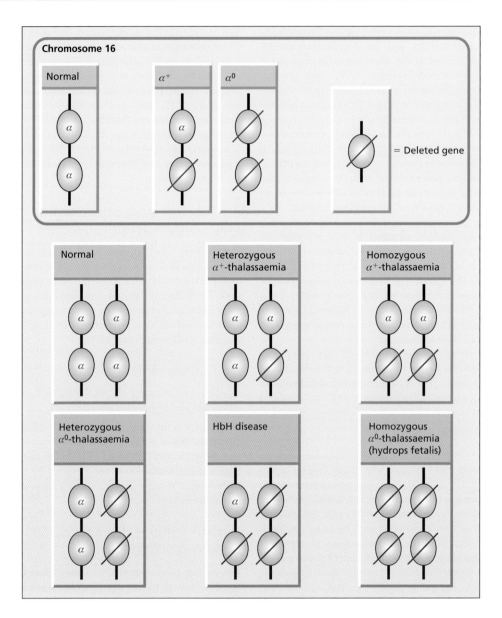

Figure 4.3 A diagram to show how the two forms of abnormal chromosome 16 (α^+ and α^0) are arranged to give the different forms of α-thalassaemia. Homozygotes for α^0-thalassaemia die from Hb Bart's hydrops fetalis syndrome.

Most patients will be transfusion independent, or require transfusions only at times of intercurrent infection. Splenomegaly is seen in most patients. (The clinical picture is therefore one of thalassaemia intermedia – see below).

Hb Bart's hydrops fetalis syndrome (deletion of all four α-globin genes)

This occurs when there is homozygosity for an α^0-thalassaemia allele. No α-chains can be formed, and the fetal β-like chain γ-globin forms tetramers known as Hb Bart's. This haemoglobin is not useful for oxygen transport and, despite the persistence of the embryonic haemoglobin Hb Portland ($\zeta_2\gamma_2$), there is intrauterine or neonatal death due to hydrops.

β-Thalassaemia

The World Health Organization estimates that 1.5% of the world's population are carriers of β-thalassaemia. The prevalence of the β-thalassaemia trait is particularly

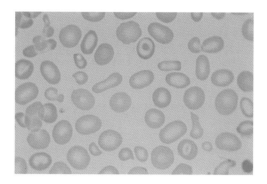

Figure 4.4 Blood film from a patient with HbH disease showing microcytosis, hypochromia, anisocytosis and poikilocytosis.

high in southern Europe (10–30%) and south-east Asia (5%), but it is also common in Africa, the Middle East, India, Pakistan and southern China. It has been suggested that the high prevalence of β-thalassaemia in these regions results from its protective effect against *Plasmodium falciparum* in heterozygotes.

While α-thalassaemia typically arises from gene deletions, β-thalassaemia usually results from a multiplicity of different single nucleotide substitutions, insertions or small deletions affecting the β-gene itself, its promoter or its upstream regulatory sequences. The prevalence of particular abnormalities varies between different ethnic groups. Analagous to the α-thalassaemias, β^0-thalassaemia describes a mutation that abolishes β-chain production from a given chromosome, while β^+-thalassaemia alleles allow some β-chain production, albeit at a reduced level. The β^0 type predominates in India and Pakistan and β^+ mutations predominate in Sardinia and Cyprus; both types are found in Greece, the Middle East and Thailand.

Heterozygous β-thalassaemia (Beta-thalassaemia trait)

Most affected subjects with beta thalassaemia trait are asymptomatic. The Hb concentration is either normal or slightly reduced, and hypochromic and microcytic red cell indices are seen. Examination of the peripheral blood film may also show characteristic red cell abnormalities such as target cells and poikilocytes. A further major clue to the diagnosis is the up-regulation of δ-globin expression. This occurs, by mechanisms yet to be fully understood, from alleles in which β-globin expression is reduced or absent. The increased δ-chains will join the normally produced α-globin chains to form HbA$_2$ ($\alpha_2\delta_2$). Typically in heterozygous β-thalassaemia HbA2 levels will be

raised above the normal range to 3.5–7.0%. Some cases also show slightly increased HbF levels, in the range of 1–5%.

Homozygous β-thalassaemia

The exact nature of the mutations affecting the β-globin cluster plus the impact of various genetic modifiers will determine the phenotype of patients with defects of β-globin on both copies of chromosome 11. In the more severe cases, marked anaemia develops between the second and twelfth months of life and patients become transfusion dependent. In other cases a more moderate anaemia is seen, presenting after the age of 1–2 years and requiring transfusion only intermittently or in the context of intercurrent infection.

Clinical classification of the thalassaemias

The molecular basis for the thalassaemias is very diverse, and even in cases where the precise molecular defect is known the impact of genetic modifiers may make it difficult to predict the exact clinical phenotype. Therefore, a clinical classification of the thalassaemias allows a description of the patient's phenotype irrespective of the exact molecular details of their underlying condition.

Thalassaemia minima describes the presence of a thalassaemic mutation that is without clinical consequences.

Thalassaemia minor describes patients with microcytosis and hypochromic red cells secondary to thalassaemia mutations, but with only mild anaemia or a normal haemoglobin. Patients who inherit a single affected allele are usually in this category.

Thalassaemia intermedia patients will also have a microcytic hypochromic anaemia, but usually of moderate degree. They will have an increased erythroid drive to maintain their haemoglobin, and will therefore have a packed bone marrow with a decreased myeloid:erythoid ratio, and extramedullary haematopoiesis, giving splenomegaly. Transfusion may be required to maintain the haemoglobin at times of additional physiological stress (e.g. during intercurrent infection), but, critically, they are normally transfusion independent. Patients in this category include some patients homozygous for mutations that reduce but do not completely obliterate β-globin expression and those with HbH disease.

Patients with *thalassaemia major* have severe anaemia and are transfusion dependent. Their increased erythroid drive leads to a packed erythroid marrow and splenomegaly. The transfusion programme is essential to avoid growth retardation and the development of bony abnormalities secondary to unchecked marrow expansion. Patients in this category are those with complete loss of β-globin expression from both copies of chromosome 11. The ongoing production of fetal haemoglobin into infancy permits these patients to survive, unlike those with complete loss of α-globin expression; but with the progressive loss of fetal haemoglobin in the first few months of life, the infant becomes profoundly anaemic and would die without transfusional support.

The clinical course and complications of thalassaemia major

While anaemia is the principal feature of thalassaemia major, the massive expansion of erythroid activity results in several complications. The development of splenomegaly and bony deformities has already been discussed, but there are also typically the general features of hypermetabolic states, such as growth retardation. Iron absorption from the gut is increased (see Chapter 2) and, in conjunction with iron loading from red cell transfusions, this contributes to marked iron overload. Iron deposition occurs in the myocardium, which can cause congestive cardiac failure and potentially fatal arrhythmias; in the liver, leading to cirrhosis; in the pancreas, causing diabetes mellitus; and in other endocrine organs, leading to delayed puberty and delay or failure in the development of secondary sexual characteristics. While untransfused patients are likely to succumb to their anaemia in the first decade of life, transfused patients have their life expectancy reduced by the development of iron overload, and controlling iron loading is therefore a key goal in the treatment of patients with thalassaemia major.

Treatment of β-thalassaemia major

Transfusions are planned to maintain the pretransfusion Hb concentration at 9–10g/dL or above, with a post-transfusion Hb concentration of 13–14 g/dL. With this treatment, thalassaemic children are able to grow and mature normally. If the spleen is considerably enlarged with evidence that it is also trapping transfused red cells and increasing transfusion requirements, splenectomy can be performed. Splenectomy may also be considered if there is thrombocytopenia or leucopenia secondary to pooling of the blood volume in the enlarged spleen.

As mentioned above, an important aspect of treatment is the reduction of tissue damage due to secondary iron overload. Until recently, this required the use of desferrioxamine, an iron chelator that could be administered only parenterally and required subcutaneous infusion treatment over several hours on five days of the week. Unsurprisingly for such a burdensome treatment, compliance can be problematic. Oral iron chelators have been made available more recently and include deferasirox (Exjade). Effective iron chelation is critical to the long-term health of patients with thalassaemia major, and may also be needed in patients with thalassaemia intermedia, due to the effects of increased iron absorption from the gut.

More radical and curative approaches have also been taken in thalassaemia major. Haemopoietic stem cell transplantation has been performed in many patients with thalassaemia major, although the limiting factor is frequently the availability of HLA-matched donors. Although the morbidity and mortality of the procedure in young patients (treated before the development of end-organ damage by iron deposition) are small, they are not negligible; the risks of the procedure therefore have to be weighed against the prospect of decades of treatment by blood transfusion and iron chelation, and a personalized treatment plan must be created for each patient. In older patients transplantation has proved less attractive an option, largely due to the higher procedure-related morbidity and mortality.

More experimental treatments include gene therapy. At least one patient with β-thalassaemia major has become transfusion independent following infusion of his own genetically modified haemopoietic stem cells, in which a functioning β-globin gene was incorporated using a lentiviral vector. While problems remain with this highly experimental technique, gene therapy remains a possible long-term goal for patients with thalassaemia major.

Genetic counselling and antenatal diagnosis of β-thalassaemia major

When a pregnant woman is found to have an abnormality in the synthesis or structure of Hb, her partner must also be investigated. If there is a risk of a serious clinical disease in the fetus, antenatal diagnosis should be offered. Antenatal diagnosis can be made early during pregnancy from an analysis of chorionic villous DNA (at 9–12 weeks) or amniocyte DNA (at 13–16 weeks), or later using DNA from blood obtained from an 18–20-week-old fetus. Newer techniques focus on the non-invasive analysis of fetal DNA in the maternal circulation.

Table 4.1 **Different clinical and haematological abnormalities associated with some structural haemoglobin variants.**

Variant	Clinical and haematological abnormalities
HbS	Recurrent painful crises (in adults) and chronic haemolytic anaemia, both related to sickling of red cells on deoxygenation
HbC	Chronic haemolytic anaemia due to reduced red cell deformability on deoxygenation; deoxygenated HbC is less soluble than deoxygenated HbA
Hb Köln, Hb Hammersmith	Spontaneous or drug-induced haemolytic anaemia due to instability of the Hb and consequent intracellular precipitation
HbM Boston, HbM Saskatoon	Cyanosis due to congenital methaemoglobinaemia as a consequence of a substitution near or in the haem pocket
Hb Chesapeake, Hb Radcliffe	Hereditary polycythaemia due to increased O_2 affinity
Hb Kansas	Anaemia and cyanosis due to decreased O_2 affinity
Hb Constant Spring, Hb Lepore, HbE	Thalassaemia-like syndrome due to decreased rate of synthesis of abnormal globin chain
Hb Indianapolis	Thalassaemia-like syndrome due to marked instability of Hb

Structural haemoglobin variants

Over 1000 abnormal haemoglobin variants have been reported, but most are rare and only a few lead to clinical or haematological manifestations. The majority of structural Hb variants are the consequence of a single-point mutation with a single amino acid substitution in the affected globin chain (e.g. HbS, HbE, HbC and HbD).

The spectrum of clinical and haematological abnormalities that may be caused by abnormal haemoglobins is summarized in Table 4.1. When the amino acid substitution results in an overall change in the charge of the haemoglobin molecule, its migration in a voltage gradient is altered and this can be demonstrated by standard electrophoretic techniques. The speed of migration is characteristic for each abnormal haemoglobin (Figure 4.5). Abnormal haemoglobin variants are now usually detected by high-performance liquid chromatography (HPLC).

The most common structural Hb variant is haemoglobin S (HbS). This globin variant, and the important clinical entity of sickle cell anaemia, are discussed in the following section.

Haemoglobin S

Sickle cell anaemia has been described as the first 'molecular disease': it was the first condition in which

a defect in a specific protein was determined to be causative (by Linus Pauling and colleagues in 1948), with the specific amino acid change being defined in 1956. A mutation in the β-globin gene results in the charged glutamic acid residue in position 6 of the nor-

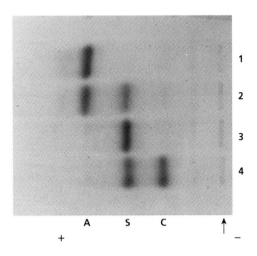

Figure 4.5 Electrophoresis of haemolysates on cellulose acetate (pH 8.5). The arrow marks the site of application of the haemolysate. (1) Normal adult. (2) Individual with sickle-cell trait; 35% of the Hb consists of HbS and most of the remainder is HbA. (3) Patient with sickle cell anaemia; most of the Hb is S and there is no A. (4) Double heterozygote for HbS and HbC. This results in a disease that is usually milder than that in homozygotes for HbS.

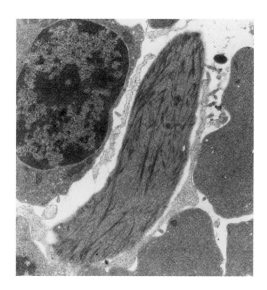

Figure 4.6 Electron micrograph of a sickled red cell from a homozygote for HbS showing fibres of polymerized deoxygenated HbS running along the long axis of the cell.

mal β-chain being replaced by an uncharged valine molecule. The interaction of sickle β-globin chains with normal α-globin chains forms HbS. When deoxygenated, HbS is much less soluble than deoxygenated HbA, and HbS molecules polymerize, eventually forming long fibres (tactoids — see Figure 4.6). These result in the deformation of the cell into the well-recognized sickle shape (Figure 4.7). Red cells from heterozygotes for HbS sickle at much lower pO$_2$ values than those from homozygotes, and do not usually sickle *in vivo*.

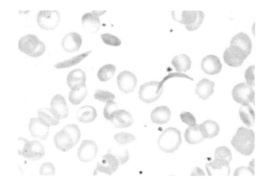

Figure 4.7 Two sickle-shaped red cells with pointed ends and some partially sickled red cells from the blood film of a patient with sickle cell anaemia (homozygote for HbS).

The gene for β^S occurs particularly in a wide area across tropical Africa, as well as in parts of the Middle East and southern India (see Figure 4.2). Its prevalence in these areas varies from very low values up to 40% of the population. In black Americans, the prevalence is 8%. The distribution of the β^S gene corresponds to areas in which falciparum malaria has been endemic; its persistence at high frequency in these areas reflects the relative resistance of heterozygotes to severe falciparum malaria during early childhood.

Sickle cell trait

Heterozygotes (one gene for normal β-globin and one for β^S) are described as having sickle cell trait. Their red cells contain between 20% and 45% HbS, the rest being mainly HbA. Heterozygotes do not have 50% HbS, mainly because mutant β-chains (β^S) have a lower affinity than normal β-chains to associate with α-chains. Individuals with sickle cell trait are usually asymptomatic. However, spontaneous haematuria may occur occasionally due to microvascular infarctions in the renal medulla. Renal papillary necrosis may rarely occur and there is often an impaired ability to concentrate urine in older individuals. The red cells do not sickle until the O$_2$ saturation falls below 40%, a level that is rarely reached in venous blood.

Sickle cell anaemia

Homozygotes for sickle β-globin are described as having sickle-cell anaemia. Their red cells contain almost exclusively HbS and no HbA; there is a small but variable percentage of fetal haemoglobin.

The cells may sickle at the O$_2$ tension normally found in venous blood. Sickled red cells then occlude the microvasculature, with poor downstream perfusion and oxygenation. They may be lysed directly in the circulation, where the resulting free haemoglobin scavenges nitric oxide; this in turn promotes vascular endothelial dysfunction and further vaso-occlusion. Sickled cells have also been shown to have abnormal interaction with endothelial cells, promoting an inflammatory reaction and inappropriate activation of the coagulation cascade. Thus, although sickling of red cells due the poor solubility of deoxygenated HbS is the ultimate basis of sickle cell anaemia, the disease is now recognized to be much more complex than the simple obstruction of the microvasculature by sickled cells. Our understanding of the pathophysiology of this condition remains far from complete.

Initially, there are cycles of sickling and reversal of sickling as the red cells are repeatedly deoxygenated and reoxygenated within the circulation. Eventually, as membrane damage accumulates, irreversibly sickled cells are formed. Both unsickled and sickled red cells containing deoxygenated HbS are less deformable than normal red cells and this results in a chronic, principally extravascular, haemolytic anaemia. The Hb usually varies between 6 and 9 g/dL, but the symptoms referable to the anaemia itself are milder than expected from the Hb levels, as HbS has a reduced affinity for O_2 (i.e. the O_2 dissociation curve is shifted to the right).

Diagnosis

Sickled cells are invariably present on the blood films of patients with HbSS (Figure 4.7). The diagnosis of HbSS is made by finding (i) a positive result with a screening test for HbS; and (ii) a peak at an appropriate position on an HPLC trace, confirmed by isoelectric focusing or haemoglobin electrophoresis. The screening tests for HbS-containing red cells are based on the decreased solubility of deoxygenated HbS; they involve the development of turbidity after addition to a lysis buffer containing a reducing agent such as sodium dithionite (sickle solubility test). Heterozygotes for HbS also give a positive result with these screening tests, but would be expected to show both HbA and HbS on HPLC/haemoglobin electrophoresis.

The clinical picture in sickle cell anaemia is highly variable (Table 4.2), reflecting the impact of genetic modifiers. Patients with hereditary persistence of fetal haemoglobin, for example, have a much milder phenotype than those patients in whom HbF is appropriately silenced. The co-inheritance of the α-thalassaemia trait, which will reduce the mean cell haemoglobin concentration, can also ameliorate the symptoms of sickle cell anaemia.

Typically, individuals with sickle cell anaemia have crises superimposed on their chronic haemolytic state, sometimes precipitated by infection, cold or dehydration, but sometimes with no obvious precipitant at all. Crises frequently take the form of acute vaso-occlusive painful episodes, which can affect any part of the body. In young children, a classic acute painful presentation is with dactylitis, or the 'hand–foot syndrome', in which there is occlusion of the nutrient arteries to the metacarpals and metatarsals (Figure 4.8) and painful swelling of the hands and feet.

Aside from painful crises, sickle cell anaemia also has wide-ranging complications that may affect any organ of the body. In the central nervous system, cerebral infarction occurs in approximately 10% of patients under the age of 20, and is a cause of significant morbidity in sickle cell patients. It has been found that children

Table 4.2 Clinical manifestations of sickle-cell anaemia.

Chronic haemolytic anaemia and consequent cholelithiasis

Splenic sequestration syndrome; rarely, hepatic sequestration

Acute chest syndrome

Cerebral infarction, TIA, intracranial haemorrhage

Widespread painful vaso-occlusive crises

Bone infarction (osteonecrosis)

Osteomyelitis (*Salmonella*, *Staphylococcus*)

Chronic leg ulcers

Priapism

Chronic pulmonary disease and pulmonary hypertension

Haematuria, proteinuria, chronic renal failure

Pregnancy: increased peripartum fetal loss, preterm births, babies small for gestational age

Aplastic crises due to parvovirus infection

Proliferative sickle retinopathy (more common in HbSC disease)

with an increased velocity of blood flow in the major cerebral vessels are at particular risk of stroke, and transcranial Doppler studies now constitute an important part of the screening of paediatric patients with sickle cell anaemia. Children with high-risk transcranial Doppler readings receive prophylactic treatment to minimize their risk of stroke (see below).

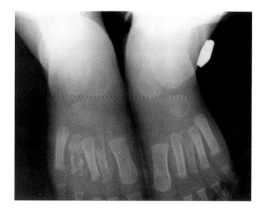

Figure 4.8 An X-ray of the feet of a child with sickle cell anaemia two weeks after the onset of hand–foot syndrome, showing necrosis of the right fourth metatarsal.

Haemorrhagic stroke may also be seen, but is commoner in older patients.

Cardio-respiratory presentations include the acute sickle chest syndrome (typically a febrile illness with dyspnoea, chest pain and radiological changes), which is the most common cause of death in adults with sickle cell anaemia. This syndrome results from a combination of pulmonary infection, infarction and sequestration and, while the clinical course is highly variable, some patients deteriorate rapidly and require intubation and ventilatory support. More chronic cardio-respiratory complications include the development of pulmonary hypertension and right heart failure, with a number of contributory factors including thromboembolism, multiple episodes of acute chest syndrome, and endothelial dysfunction from nitric oxide scavenging.

As with all chronic haemolytic anaemias, there is an increase in the incidence of pigment gallstones. Additional hepatic complications can include vaso-occlusion of the hepatic sinusoids, which can result in marked cholestasis. Renal complications include renal papillary necrosis as a result of infarction. Renal failure is thought to develop in up to a quarter of patients with HbSS and is caused by a combination of cortical and medullary infarction, glomerular sclerosis, tubular damage and infection. Priapism is another common problem.

Young children can develop potentially life-threatening acute splenic sequestration – a crisis caused by the rapid and extensive trapping of red cells in the spleen, leading to profound anaemia, massive splenomegaly, reduced blood volume and hypovolaemic shock. Repeated splenic infarcts lead to functional hyposplenism, with an increased risk of infection, particularly due to encapsulated organisms. Infection is the biggest cause of mortality in paediatric sickle cell patients, particularly as a consequence of fulminant bacterial infections, but an increased risk of infection remains problematic throughout life.

In terms of musculoskeletal and skin complications, patients may suffer from larger infarcts affecting the bones, with avascular necrosis of the femoral head being a potential complication. Osteomyelitis is another recognized complication and is classically found to be due to *Salmonella* Typhi. Chronic leg ulcers are often seen (Figure 4.9) and can be very difficult to treat.

A proliferative sickle retinopathy may develop and can lead to blindness from vitreous haemorrhage and retinal detachment; retinopathy is more common in compound heterozygotes for HbS and HbC (i.e. in HbSC disease) than in sickle cell anaemia, and results from hypoxaemic conditions downstream of occluded vessels.

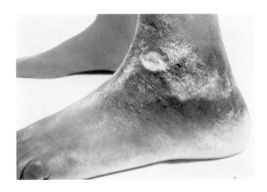

Figure 4.9 A chronic leg ulcer with increased pigmentation of the surrounding skin in a woman with sickle cell anaemia.

Aplastic crises due to parvovirus infection may occur (p. 28), as may an exacerbation of the anaemia due to secondary folic acid deficiency (p. 20).

Treatment

The principles of the management of sickle cell anaemia include:

- Management of the increased infection risk by immunization with pneumococcal, *Haemophilus influenzae* type b (Hib) and meningococcal vaccine, plus treatment with prophylactic penicillin. This is particularly critical for children, but continues lifelong. Non-immune patients should also receive hepatitis B vaccine in case multiple transfusions are required.
- Administration of folic acid daily to prevent secondary folate deficiency.
- Avoidance of factors precipitating painful crises such as dehydration, hypoxia, circulatory stasis.
- Active treatment for bacterial infections that may precipitate or have precipitated crises.
- Treatment of painful crises with oral or intravenous fluids and analgesics, including opiates when necessary.
- Early detection of the acute chest syndrome (blood gas measurements and chest X-ray), with the administration of oxygen and respiratory support where appropriate. Exchange transfusions are often needed to lower the patient's HbS levels and limit ongoing sickling.
- Blood transfusion when necessary. Careful top-up transfusion may be indicated for sequestration and aplastic crises, and exchange transfusions are useful in certain situations – particularly in severe acute chest syndrome, in priapism and in cases where there is evidence of neurological damage.

Exchange transfusion followed by a chronic transfusion programme may also be initiated in children considered to be at highest risk of stroke. When transcranial Doppler studies suggest a high risk of stroke, a regular transfusion programme that suppresses the patient's own erythroid drive will reduce the HbS content of blood, and this has been shown in clinical trials to have a major impact on reducing the incidence of stroke. A similar programme may also be initiated in patients of any age who suffer particularly frequent crises. As in the case of thalassaemia major, patients who are regularly transfused for prolonged periods (>1-2 years) must receive iron chelators to prevent iron overload. Transfusion may also be required during pregnancy in patients with frequent crises or a poor obstetric history.

In patients having frequent severe crises (three or more per year), strategies other than transfusion plus iron chelation include agents to reinduce the expression of fetal haemoglobin. The fetal γ-globin chains cannot be incorporated into the polymerized sickle haemoglobin, such that the presence of haemoglobin F is able to inhibit the sickling process. Sickle cell patients with co-inherited inappropriate expression of γ-globin after infancy (known as hereditary persistence of fetal haemoglobin, HPFH) have a much milder phenotype than those in whom fetal globin is silenced normally. Much research effort has therefore gone into understanding the mechanisms by which fetal globin is silenced (see Box 4.1), with a view to its therapeutic reactivation. The current pharmacological intervention to try to elevate HbF expression is long-term therapy with the ribonucleotide reductase inhibitor hydroxycarbamide; this increases the synthesis of HbF to a limited extent by means that are incompletely understood, and indeed modes of action other than HbF induction have been proposed to explain its therapeutic benefits. Whatever the true basis of its effect, it can yield a significant reduction in the frequency of crises, and also significantly reduces mortality in patients with more than three vaso-occlusive crises per year.

Curative strategies do exist. As with thalassaemia major, bone marrow transplantation is currently the only curative treatment, though it is relatively rarely performed. Patients with a suitably severe phenotype must be identified prior to the onset of organ damage; consequently most transplants have been undertaken in children, with the best results seen in those with matched sibling donors. Typical overall survival rates are 90-97%, with event-free survival being near 85%. The potential risks of the procedure need to be weighed carefully against the implications of chronic disease for each young patient when deciding on an appropriate treatment strategy.

Prognosis

There is a high infant mortality rate, especially when the quality of health care or compliance with advice is poor. With the use of prophylactic penicillin V (from two months old), childhood deaths due to pneumococcal sepsis have been substantially reduced. In adults, the acute chest syndrome is a common cause of death, with mortality rates between 5% and 10%. Even with optimal current treatment, the life expectancy for patients with sickle cell anaemia is still reduced to approximately 50 years.

Haemoglobins E and C

There are many haemoglobin variants other than HbS with clinical consequences. Among the commonest are HbE and HbC, both of which result from single amino acid substitutions in the β-chains.

Box 4.1: Reactivating silenced fetal haemoglobin

The β-globinopathies present a major burden of morbidity and mortality worldwide. All present clinically as the normal haemoglobin 'switch' from HbF to HbA takes place in the first few months after birth; patients with hereditary persistence of fetal haemoglobin are therefore largely protected from the most severe clinical manifestations.

The possibility of reactivating the normal γ-globin gene alongside the defective β-globin gene has long been considered an attractive therapeutic option. Yet, as with all genes, the details of how its expression is activated and silenced in a developmental stage-specific manner remain poorly understood.

A significant step forward was made in 2008 with the discovery of the role of BCL11a, a DNA-binding protein. Sequence variants in the gene for BCL11a were found to be frequently implicated in patients with hereditary persistence of fetal hemoglobin, and subsequent work demonstrated that high levels of BCL11a were found only in mature red cells. Moreover, the experimental down-regulation of BCL11a is able to reinstate high levels of HbF production, with clinically relevant amelioration of the haematological phenotype in animal models of sickle cell anaemia. Work is underway to find a method of exploiting this finding for clinical benefit. Meanwhile, agents such as hydroxycarbamide, which can achieve modest elevations of HbF synthesis, are widely used in the treatment of sickle cell anaemia.

HbE is a structural variant of β-globin in which a missense mutation creates a new splice site at the end of the first intron/exon boundary. Patients with HbE therefore have a reduction in normally spliced β-globin mRNA, with subsequent reduction in the amount of β-globin produced from the affected allele – rather like a form of β-thalassaemia. Heterozygotes have about 20–30% HbE, are asymptomatic and are usually not anaemic, although they do have a low MCV consistent with the thalassaemia-like pathophysiology. Homozygotes are characterized by mild anaemia, a low MCV and many circulating target cells. The main clinical significance of this globin variant, however, is its co-inheritance with β-thalassaemia. As HbE is very common in south-east Asia (being found in about 50% of the population in some parts of Thailand), compound heterozygosity for Eβ-thalassaemia is not unusual. Such patients have highly variable clinical presentations, but the more severely affected have a thalassaemia major phenotype and need long-term transfusion programmes.

HbC is the consequence of a glutamine to lysine substitution in the β-globin chain, producing a positively charged haemoglobin molecule. When co-inherited with a sickle allele, the resulting HbSC gives a sickling phenotype, although with some specific features (such as a more marked propensity to proliferative retinopathy). HbC is also seen in homozygosity; here the haemoglobin does not polymerize as with HbSS, but can crystallize, with a resulting reduction in the flexibility of the red cell and a reduction in its survival. Abnormalities of potassium handling within HbCC red cells also contribute to the pheno-

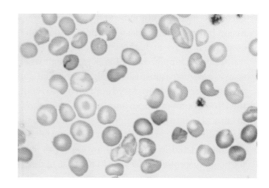

Figure 4.10 Target cells and irregularly contracted cells in the blood film of a homozygote for HbC.

type. Homozygotes have a mild anaemia, low MCV, splenomegaly and many target cells in their blood film (Figure 4.10), while heterozygotes tend to be clinically asymptomatic. HbC is found in patients of West African origin, where the incidence may be as high as 7% of the population in Nigeria and 22% in northern Ghana.

While HbS, HbE and HbC are among the commonest structural defects in the globins, many others exist, each with its own impact on the normal structure and function of haemoglobin. An understanding of the molecular nature of these disorders has been crucial to appreciating their pathophysiology and is likely to be of benefit in developing effective therapies in the future.

5

Conditions associated with white cell abnormalities

Learning objectives

✓ To understand the meaning of the terms leucopenia, neutropenia, leucocytosis, lymphopenia and lymphocytosis

✓ To understand the significance of neutropenic sepsis and the importance of early identification and treatment

✓ To know the common disorders associated with atypical lymphocytes in the blood, particularly Epstein–Barr virus (EBV) infection

---

Leucopenia

The terms 'leucopenia' and 'neutropenia' are used to describe a reduction in the total white cell count and neutrophil count, respectively, to values below their normal ranges. The term 'lymphopenia' is used when the lymphocyte count is subnormal.

Neutropenia

Neutrophils are highly motile cells that are required to maintain the integrity of mucosal surfaces and prevent overwhelming bacterial infection (see Chapter 1). There is a substantial risk of serious infection when the neutrophil count falls below 0.5×10^9/L. The first symptom of neutropenia is sore throat (mucositis) and fever. Breakdown of the gastrointestinal mucosa may lead to Gram-negative septicaemia, hypotension and death (*neutropenic sepsis*). The management of neutropenic sepsis requires rapid assessment: urgent investigations including blood cultures and immediate use of intravenous antibiotics and adequate hydration. If the fever persists, a programme of planned progressive therapy is used (Figure 5.1). Patients with prolonged neutropenia are particularly prone to develop fungal infections, notably *Candida* and *Aspergillus*. *Candida* species usually affect the mouth and other mucosal surfaces, whereas *Aspergillus* species tend to cause invasive pulmonary disease.

Selective neutropenia (neutropenia without other cytopenias) may occur in a large number of conditions (Table 5.1). Cytotoxic drugs and radiotherapy cause a predictable neutropenia. Some combination chemotherapy regimens can lead to predictable neutropenia lasting days to weeks. Patients undergoing such treatment who become febrile require support with broad spectrum intravenous antibiotics and antifungal agents based on planned progressive therapy, outlined above. Other drugs (Table 5.1), for example carbimazole, used to treat hyperthyroidism, and some antimalarial drugs are associated with idiosyncratic neutropenia. Patients taking these drugs should be warned about the remote but possible risk of neutropenia and advised to stop the drug should they develop a sore throat or fever.

Haematology Lecture Notes, Ninth edition. C.S.R. Hatton, N.C. Hughes-Jones, D. Hay and D. Keeling. © 2013 John Wiley & Sons, Ltd.
Published 2013 by John Wiley & Sons, Ltd.

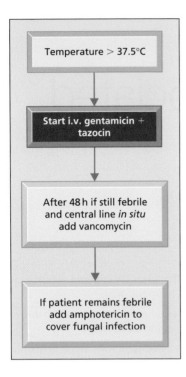

Figure 5.1 Planned progressive therapy for febrile patients with neutropenia (<0.5 × 10⁹ L).

Leucocytosis

An increase in the total white cell count is described as a leucocytosis. The term 'neutrophil leucocytosis' is used to describe an absolute increase in the total number of neutrophils in the peripheral blood (also known as neutrophilia). Eosinophilia is the term used to describe an absolute increase in the number of eosinophils. Similarly, basophilia is the term used to describe an absolute increase in the basophil count. Monocytosis describes an increase in the absolute monocyte count.

Neutrophil leucocytosis

The causes of neutrophil leucocytosis are shown in Table 5.2. Bacterial infection is an important cause, but many varied insults will elevate the neutrophil count. In addition, metamyelocytes and small numbers of myelocytes may be present in severe infection – 'shift to the left'. Neutrophils may show toxic granulation (Figure 5.2), or Döhle bodies (Figure 5.3) or both. Toxic granules are abnormally coarse, reddish violet (azurophilic) granules, which are diffusely distributed throughout the cytoplasm. Döhle bodies are 1–2 μm long, pale greyish blue cytoplasmic inclusions (Romanowsky stain). A 'shift to the left',

---

Table 5.1 The causes of selective neutropenia.

Physiological
Neutropenia in people of Afro-Caribbean ancestry

Certain drugs
Anti-inflammatory drugs: indomethacin, oxyphenbutazone, phenylbutazone, sodium aurothiomalate

Antibacterial drugs: chloramphenicol, co-trimoxazole (sulphamethoxazole–trimethoprim), other sulphonamides

Some anticonvulsants, oral hypoglycaemic agents, antithyroid drugs, antimalarial drugs, tranquillizers, antidepressants and antihistamines

Infections
Bacterial: overwhelming pyogenic infections, brucellosis, typhoid, miliary tuberculosis

Some viral, protozoal and fungal infections

Immune neutropenia
Systemic lupus erythematosus (SLE), Felty's syndrome, autoimmune neutropenia, neonatal alloimmune neutropenia, aminopyrine-induced agranulocytosis

Miscellaneous
Hypothyroidism, hypopituitarism, cyclical neutropenia, familial benign chronic neutropenia

---

Table 5.2 The causes of neutrophil leucocytosis.

Physiological
Neonates, exercise, pregnancy, parturition, lactation

Pathological
Acute infections: especially by pyogenic bacteria

Acute inflammation not caused by infections: surgery, burns, infarcts, crush injuries, rheumatoid arthritis, myositis, vasculitis

Acute haemorrhage and acute haemolysis

Metabolic: uraemia, diabetic ketoacidosis, gout, acute thyrotoxicosis

Non-haematological malignancies: carcinoma, melanoma

Lymphoma

Chronic myeloproliferative disorders: chronic myeloid leukaemia, polycythaemia vera, myelofibrosis

Drugs: adrenaline, corticosteroids, G-CSF and GM-CSF

Miscellaneous: convulsions, paroxysmal tachycardia, electric shock, postneutropenic rebound neutrophilia, postsplenectomy

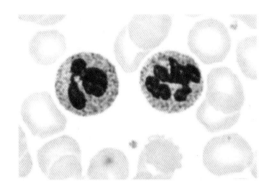

Figure 5.2 Toxic granulation in two neutrophils from a patient with an infection.

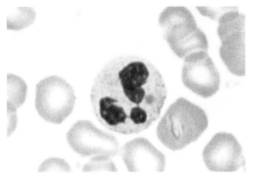

Figure 5.3 Round, pale blue Döhle body near the nucleus of a neutrophil from a patient with extensive burns. Döhle bodies may also be oval or rod shaped and are more frequently seen at the periphery than at the centre of the cell.

toxic granulation and Döhle bodies reflect accelerated neutrophil production and may be seen not only in acute infection but also in non-infective inflammatory states (e.g. severe burns), in normal pregnancy and in patients with various malignant neoplasms.

The neutrophil leucocytosis seen with steroid administration and after exercise is caused by a rapid shift of neutrophils from the marginated to the circulating granulocyte pool.

Abnormalities of granulocyte morphology and function

There are a number of inherited conditions causing abnormalities in granulocyte morphology or function or both. The essential features of some of these are summarized in Table 5.3. The most common acquired abnormalities of neutrophil morphology include 'shift to the left', hypersegmentation of the nucleus (p. 22), toxic granulation, Döhle bodies, hypogranularity and the acquired Pelger–Huët anomaly (see myelodysplasia, Chapter 11).

Eosinophilia

Eosinophilia is usually caused by allergic disorders or parasitic infestation. Asthma, eczema and drugs are the commonest causes, but there are many others, some of which are listed in Table 5.4.

Basophilia

Basophilia is an uncommon finding and should raise the possibility of a myeloid haematological malignancy such as chronic myeloid leukaemia or myelodysplasia. Other causes include myxoedema and hypersensitivity reactions.

Table 5.3 Some inherited abnormalities of neutrophil morphology or function or both.

Condition	Inheritance, prevalence	Characteristics
Pelger–Huët anomaly	Autosomal dominant 1:1000–10,000	Heterozygotes have bilobed spectacle-like neutrophil nuclei, homozygotes have round or oval neutrophil nuclei; asymptomatic
Neutrophil myeloperoxidase deficiency	Autosomal recessive 1:2000	Detected during automated differential counting based on cytochemistry; usually asymptomatic
Chediak–Higashi syndrome	Autosomal recessive	Giant granules in leucocytes, neutropenia, thrombocytopenia, partial albinism, hepatosplenomegaly, death in infancy or early childhood from infection and haemorrhage
Chronic granulomatous disease	Majority X linked, some autosomal recessive	Normal neutrophil morphology, inability to kill ingested micro-organisms due to absence of cytochrome b_{558} or other components of the respiratory chain leading to impaired superoxide generation, recurrent granulomatous lesions from early childhood

<table>
<tr><td colspan="1">

Table 5.4 The causes of eosinophilia.

Parasitic infestations: filariasis, hookworm, ascariasis, strongyloidiasis, schistosomiasis, toxocariasis, trichinosis, hydatid cyst, scabies

Allergic disorders: bronchial asthma, hayfever, allergic vasculitis, Stevens–Johnson syndrome, drug sensitivity (e.g. chlorpromazine, penicillin, sulphonamides)

Recovery from acute infection

Skin diseases: eczema, psoriasis, pemphigus, dermatitis herpetiformis

Pulmonary eosinophilia: Loeffler's syndrome (pulmonary infiltration with eosinophilia)

Polyarteritis nodosa

Chronic myeloid leukaemia, eosinophilic leukaemia (rare)

Other malignant diseases: Hodgkin lymphoma, angioimmunoblastic lymphoma, carcinoma (usually with metastases)

Idiopathic hypereosinophilic syndrome

</td></tr>
</table>

Monocytosis

A high monocyte count is seen in many inflammatory disorders and malignant states. A high monocyte count is also found in chronic myelomonocytic leukaemia, one of the myelodysplastic disorders (see Chapter 11).

Lymphocytosis and lymphopenia

An increase in the blood lymphocyte count is called a *lymphocytosis*. This is defined as a lymphocyte count greater than 4.0×10^9/L. *Lymphopenia* refers to a decrease in the number of circulating lymphocytes and is defined as a total lymphocyte count below 1×10^9/L. In normal blood most lymphocytes are CD4+ T cells. Important causes of lymphocytopenia include acquired immune deficiency syndrome (AIDS), radiotherapy, chemotherapy and steroid therapy. A transient low lymphocyte count is often found in patients with severe infection.

Transient lymphocytosis

The morphological features of lymphocytes enable the distinction between reactive and malignant causes. The most common cause of reactive lymphocytosis is infectious mononucleosis (see below).

Lymphocytosis may be associated with other viral infections such as cytomegalovirus (CMV), hepatitis and human immunodeficiency virus (HIV; early stages). Whooping cough (*Bordetella pertussis*) is an important cause of lymphocytosis in children.

Persistent lymphocytosis

Persistent lymphocytosis is suggestive of an underlying lymphoproliferative disorder and requires further characterization. There are benign causes, but in older persons the most common cause is B-cell chronic lymphocytic leukaemia. The profile of antigens expressed by cells can be determined by the technique of *flow cytometry*. The antigen profile of lymphocytes allows differentiation between malignant and benign conditions and also allows characterization of individual cells into B- and T-cell subtypes.

Flow cytometry: A technique for identification of cells in suspension

Flow cytometry is a technique used to characterize cells, usually in the peripheral blood or in bone marrow aspirate samples. It is a method that allows the detection of specific antigens on the cell surface or, if the cell is made permeable, in its cytoplasm and nucleus. This is achieved by measuring fluorescence and light scatter of cells as they flow in a coaxial stream through a beam of intense light. The fluorescence generated may be 'self-generated' autofluorescence, due to cytochromes and other intracellular components, or may arise because the cells have been prelabelled with fluorochromes conjugated to antigen-binding antibodies. It is this latter technique that permits the detection of specific cell surface antigens. Most flow cytometers use an argon laser to excite fluorochromes such as fluorescein isothiocyanate (FITC, green), phycoerythrin (PE, orange) and peridinin chlorophyll protein (PerCP, red), which are bound to cell surface antigens. The different emission spectra of the fluorochromes allow cells labelled with FITC to be distinguished from cells labelled with PE or PerCP (Figure 5.4) and this in turn enables cells carrying specific antigens to be defined.

The deflection of the laser beam by the cell also gives information about the size and granularity of the cell. Forward scatter of light relates to the size of a cell, whereas side scatter (SSC) relates to the

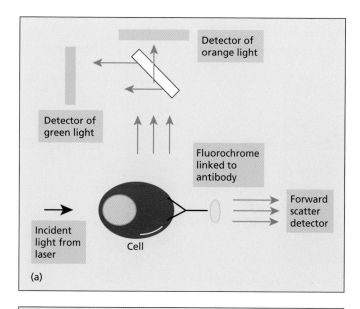

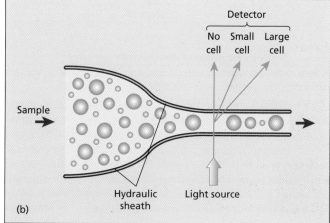

Figure 5.4 (a) Schematic diagram to illustrate general principles of flow cytometry. (b) Schematic diagram showing how cells are presented to a laser light beam by hydrodynamic focusing.

granularity of the cell. Figure 5.5 shows flow cytometry performed on a normal bone marrow incubated with anti-CD45 antibody labelled with the fluorochromes PerCP (CD45 is an antigen present on most haemopoietic cells apart from nucleated red cells, some blasts cells and plasma cells). It demonstrates the ability to separate different populations of cells within the bone marrow sample.

Infectious mononucleosis

This is a syndrome characterized by the appearance of reactive lymphocytes in the peripheral blood caused by infection (Figure 5.6). The commonest causative agent is the EBV. Other agents include *Toxoplasma gondii*, CMV and HIV.

EBV infection

EBV infection is caused by close mucosal contact (e.g. kissing a carrier). The virus infects the respiratory epithelium causing pharyngitis, often with a significant exudate on the tonsillar bed. The virus enters the blood leading to lymphadenopathy, fever and hepatosplenomegaly. Liver function tests may be abnormal. The illness is usually self-limiting, but can lead to persistent lassitude and fatigue. Patients given amoxycillin may develop a florid rash that is almost diagnostic in this clinical setting.

A characteristic feature of this illness is the development of antibodies capable of agglutinating red cells of other species – horse red cells or sheep red cells. Non-specific antibodies can be absorbed out using guinea-pig kidney cells, allowing the

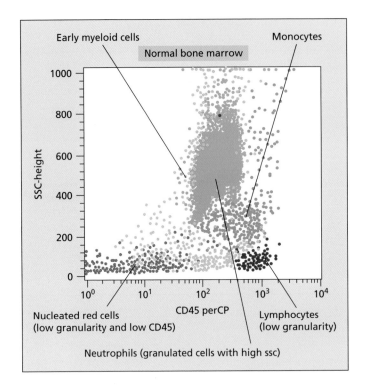

Early myeloid cells

Monocytes

Normal bone marrow

Nucleated red cells
(low granularity and low CD45)

CD45 perCP

Lymphocytes
(low granularity)

Neutrophils (granulated cells with high ssc)

Figure 5.5 Flow cytometry of normal bone marrow after incubating normal bone marrow cells with PerCP-labelled anti-CD45 antibody.

specific antibodies to be titrated against sheep red cells; this is the basis of the Paul–Bunnell test. The monospot test uses a similar agglutination reaction for the detection of heterophile antibodies against horse red blood cells. When positive, the monospot test is highly suggestive of infectious mononucleosis caused by EBV. It is also well known that some patients develop autoimmune complications such as autoimmune haemolytic anaemia and immune thrombocytopenia.

The EBV virus, having been shed from the pharyngeal mucosa, infects B-lymphocytes, causing them to proliferate. This is followed by activation of T cells, mainly CD8+ cytotoxic T cells, which control the B-cell proliferation. The 'reactive' or atypical lymphocytes characteristic of this condition consist mainly of these T cells. Infected B cells harbouring EBV persist throughout life. Asymptomatic carriers periodically shed virus from the pharynx, thereby ensuring that the virus is passed on to non-immune persons. Patients who receive immunosuppressive therapy following renal, heart/lung or bone marrow transplantation may lose the T-cell control necessary to control the EBV-infected B cells. The resulting B-cell lymphoproliferation may involve lymph nodes or extranodal sites, resulting in a condition known as a post-transplant lymphoproliferative disorder or PTLD.

Infection and immunity

Virus infection

EBV is transmitted via saliva and establishes replicative infection within cells of the oropharynx, where it expresses lytic cycle proteins. It goes on to establish

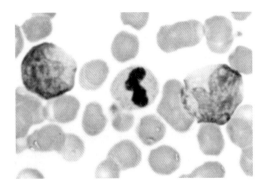

Figure 5.6 Two atypical mononuclear cells (reactive lymphocytes) and a neutrophil from a patient with glandular fever. Although the atypical mononuclear cells are similar in size to the monocyte in Figure 1.3, their cytoplasm is much more basophilic and not vacuolated.

latent infection within B cells (Figure 5.7). During the primary phase of infection all the EBV latent proteins are expressed within B cells (latency III programme of gene transcription). Following primary infection the number of infected B cells falls and expression of the viral latent proteins is down-regulated (latency I programme of gene transcription). In this form the virus can evade the host's immune response and the infection is therefore persistent. Periodic reactivation of EBV may occur, resulting in low-level virus replication in the oropharynx, virus shedding in saliva and transmission to other hosts.

Immune response

Primary infection stimulates a vigorous immune response with the expansion of CD8+ T cells specific for the EBV lytic cycle and latent proteins, and a smaller expansion of CD4+ T cells. As primary infection is controlled, the number of EBV-specific T cells falls, although a significant proportion of the T-cell pool

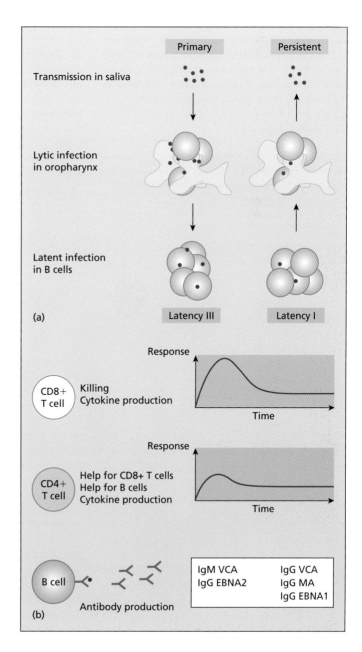

Figure 5.7 Features of EBV infection and the resulting immune response. IgM antibody to VCA is diagnostic of a recent or continuing infection. *Notes:* VCA – viral capsid antigen; EBNA – Epstein–Barr nuclear antigen; MA – membrane antigen.

remains committed to recognition of EBV. During primary infection the humoral response includes IgM antibodies specific for the viral capsid antigens (VCA) and IgG antibodies specific for the nuclear antigen, EBNA2. Neutralizing IgG antibodies, specific for a membrane antigen (MA), gp350 and IgG antibodies specific for a different nuclear antigen, EBNA1, arise later in the course of infection.

CMV infection

CMV infection usually causes a milder pharyngitis, but with a higher fever and greater splenomegaly than is found in EBV mononucleosis. The importance of CMV is in immunocompromised persons, most notably in the post-transplant setting where an absence of controlling T cells can lead to life-threatening complications such as CMV pneumonitis.

Toxoplasmosis

Toxoplasmosis often produces prominent lymphadenopathy. Fever in this condition may be absent. The finding of IgM toxoplasma antibodies is diagnostic.

HIV

HIV can present with very many different haematological manifestations, but among these is a 'mononucleosis-like' syndrome. Autoimmune haemolytic anaemia, immune thrombocytopenia and thrombotic thrombocytopenic purpura may also occur in patients with HIV.

Leucoerythroblastic reaction

The characteristic feature is the presence of nucleated red cells as well as immature white cells (mainly myelocytes) in the peripheral blood film. The finding is important, as it may be seen when the bone marrow is infiltrated with malignant cells, either haematological or non-haematological. A bone marrow aspirate and trephine biopsy may establish the diagnosis. Other causes include hypoxia and sepsis.

6

Structure and function of lymphoid tissue

Learning objectives

✓ To understand the components of the immune system

✓ To have a basic understanding of the structure of lymph nodes

✓ To know that it is immunoglobulin gene rearrangement that defines a B cell

✓ To know that it is T-cell receptor (TCR) gene rearrangement that defines a T cell

✓ To understand that malignant disorders derive from their recognizable normal counterparts

Lymphocytes can be divided into three main classes of effector cell: B-lymphocytes, T-lymphocytes and natural killer (NK) cells, all of which derive from precursor cells in the bone marrow (Figure 6.1).

B cells are the effector cells of *humoral immunity (antibody production)* and are thought to arise in the bone marrow, where they begin life as a blast cell and mature in peripheral lymphoid tissue (e.g. lymph nodes, gut and bone marrow), to become antibody-producing *plasma cells*. This maturation involves rearrangement and mutation of their immunoglobulin genes, allowing expression of surface and secreted immunoglobulin with a wide range of antigen-binding specificities.

T cells are the effector cells of *cell-mediated immunity*. Precursors of T cells migrate to the thymus, where they develop into CD4 (helper) and CD8 (suppressor/cytotoxic) cells, before migrating to other lymphoid organs, including the spleen and bone marrow.

NK cells mediate *natural killer cell function*. These cells lack B- or T-cell markers and were previously referred to as null cells. They have a characteristic morphology, being generally larger than other lymphocytes and having small granules in their cytoplasm ('large granular lymphocytes') (Figure 1.8).

Lymph node structure

Lymph nodes contain densely packed T- and B-lymphocytes, organized in a manner that allows the presentation of antigen to produce an effective immune response. In addition to having a blood supply, lymph nodes receive 'afferent' lymphatic vessels, which drain antigen-rich lymph from the tissues. Within the unstimulated lymph node, resting B cells are organized into structures called *primary follicles* (Figure 6.2). When exposed to antigen (e.g. from micro-organisms), these structures enlarge and *germinal centres* develop, comprising proliferating B cells lying within a meshwork of 'follicular dendritic cells'. Surrounding the follicles there are sheets of lymphocytes, which become increasingly rich in T cells towards the lymph node medulla. The medulla contains different types of lymphocytes, including plasma cells.

Haematology Lecture Notes, Ninth edition. C.S.R. Hatton, N.C. Hughes-Jones, D. Hay and D. Keeling. © 2013 John Wiley & Sons, Ltd.
Published 2013 by John Wiley & Sons, Ltd.

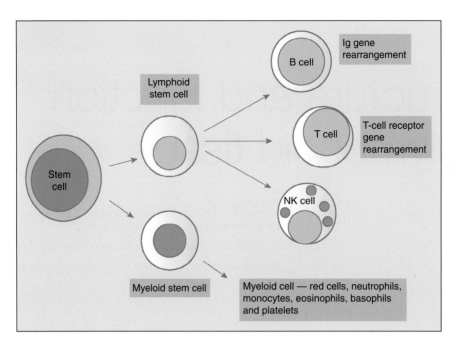

Figure 6.1 The derivation of B cells, T cells and NK cells from stem cells.

Other lymphoid tissue

Lymphoid tissue is found in many sites other than lymph nodes. These sites include tissues directly exposed to external pathogens (e.g. the respiratory and gastrointestinal tracts) and also 'central sites' such as the bone marrow and spleen. Plasma cells are found in many lymphoid tissues, particularly at sites where they can secrete immunoglobulin into the circulation or mucous secretions (e.g. into the respiratory or gastrointestinal tracts).

Immunoglobulin structure and gene rearrangement

The defining feature of B-cell development is the production of immunoglobulin with a wide range of antibody specificities. Immunoglobulins are made up of two identical heavy chains and two identical light chains (either κ or λ) (Figure 6.3). The five major classes of immunoglobulin – IgA, IgG, IgM, IgD and IgE – are defined by their heavy chains (α, γ, μ, δ and ε). The two heavy chains and two light chains are held together in a Y-shaped structure. The amino terminal portions of the heavy and light chains are known as 'variable' regions (V_H or V_L),

since differences in their amino acid sequence create unique antigen-binding sites, each of which can recognize a different epitope. In contrast, the carboxy terminal regions are the 'constant' regions (C_H or C_L), because their structure is similar for all immunoglobulins of the same class. The enzyme papain cleaves the immunoglobulin molecule into an Fc fragment consisting of the carboxy terminal regions of the heavy chain and two Fab fragments containing the antigen-binding site. A number of cell types possess Fc receptors that can bind the Fc portion of immunoglobulin molecules.

Human plasma contains all types of immunoglobulin, but IgG is present at the highest concentration. IgA is the second commonest type of immunoglobulin and is found at mucosal surfaces in the gut and the respiratory system. IgM represents only 6% of the immunoglobulin found in plasma and is the antibody most commonly produced during a primary immune response. IgM has a very large molecular weight (ca. 900,000 kDa) and is pentameric in structure. The high molecular weight of IgM can be very relevant in disorders such as Waldenstrom's macroglobulinaemia, where large amounts of secreted monoclonal protein can cause a considerable increase in blood viscosity.

Light chains

These are low molecular weight proteins (23 kDa) and are present in a $\kappa{:}\lambda$ ratio of 2:1. The κ gene is situated

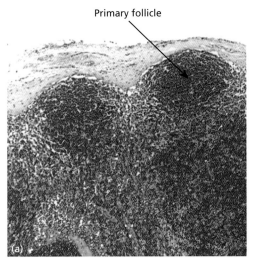

Primary follicle

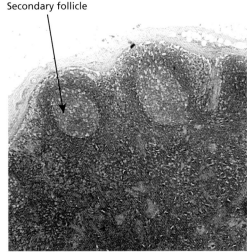

Secondary follicle

(a)

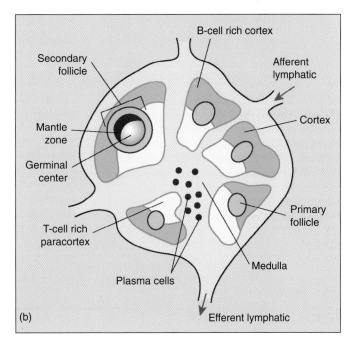

B-cell rich cortex

Secondary follicle

Afferent lymphatic

Mantle zone

Cortex

Germinal center

T-cell rich paracortex

Primary follicle

Medulla

Plasma cells

Efferent lymphatic

(b)

Figure 6.2 (a) Histological section through a lymph node and (b) drawing of a stylized lymph node.

on chromosome 2, while the λ gene is located on chromosome 22.

Heavy chains

The immunoglobulin heavy chain gene complex is located on chromosome 14. It consists of 100–200 heavy chain variable genes (V_H), at least 24 diversity genes, 6 junctional minigenes and exons that encode the heavy chain constant regions characteristic of each class (Figure 6.4).

Antibody diversity

Immunoglobulin gene rearrangement is the mechanism by which a single variable gene (V_H or V_L) in either a heavy or light chain gene complex is juxtaposed to genes encoding the constant region (C_H or C_L), generating differences from one immunoglobulin molecule to another in antigen-binding specificities (Figure 6.4). Diversity is increased by the introduction of randomly generated sequences, as well as by mutations within the variable regions. In consequence,

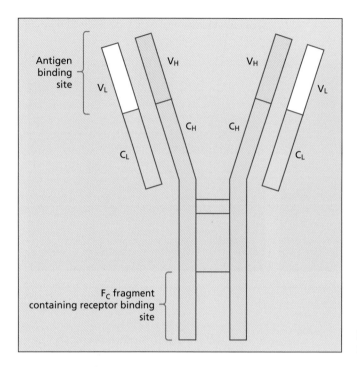

Figure 6.3 Schematic model of an IgG molecule.

a B-cell clone can synthesize immunoglobulin molecules with unique antigen-binding sites. It may be added that at different stages of differentiation, a single B cell can synthesize heavy chains with different constant regions but with the same variable regions and thus antigen specificity. Thus a B cell can start by expressing IgM but following antigen binding can produce IgG, IgA or IgE.

B-cell selection and maturation

B cells arising from progenitor cells in the bone marrow make their way to the germinal centre of lymphoid tissue, where they encounter antigen already bound to dendritic cells. If the surface immunoglobulin (sIg) on the B cells binds this antigen, the cross-linking provides a survival signal. Otherwise the B cells undergo apoptosis, a process that ensures

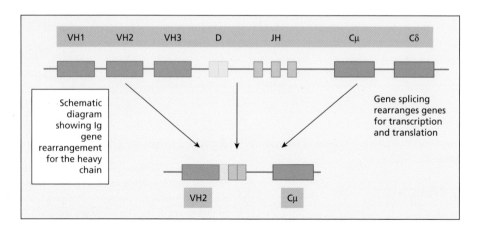

Figure 6.4 A diagram illustrating gene rearrangement enabling antigen-binding diversity. During differentiation, a single B cell can synthesize heavy chains with different constant regions coupled to the same variable region. The T-cell receptor (TCR) undergoes gene rearrangement in a very similar way in T cells. *Notes:* C – constant region gene; D – diversity gene; JH – joining sequence; V$_H$ – variable gene.

selection of 'useful' B cells, which become memory B cells and plasma cells.

T-lymphocyte antigen receptors

The antigen receptor on T cells (*T-cell receptor* or TCR) is formed from two polypeptide chains, usually α and β and less commonly γ and δ. TCR molecules are very comparable in structure to immunoglobulin molecules and the diversity in their binding sites results from a similar process (i.e. the rearrangement of variable and constant region genes). Interaction of the TCR and a binding ligand results in T-cell activation and proliferation.

During differentiation, T cells migrate from the bone marrow to the thymus, where they encounter major histocompatibility complex (MHC) class I molecules on the thymic epithelium. Any T cells that fail to recognize these molecules will die by apoptosis and the same fate awaits cells that bind with very high affinity. As a consequence, the T cells that emerge from the thymus all carry TCRs with an intermediate affinity for 'self' MHC molecules. This ensures that they will subsequently continuously bind to (and disengage from) self-MHC molecules. However, if alteration of the MHC molecule by the presence of a peptide (e.g. from a virus) increases the affinity of TCR binding, the cell presenting the peptide with the MHC molecule will become the target for specific recognition and killing.

Natural killer cells

NK cells differ from T cells in that they do not express TCRs, but they are nevertheless capable of mediating cell lysis. This is achieved through surface receptors that suppress NK activity when they engage MHC molecules on a cell. However, the absence of MHC molecules on a cell removes this inhibition and the NK cells then initiate cytotoxic destruction of the target cell.

NK cells express FcγRIIIA (CD16) – a receptor that recognizes antibody on the surface of a cell – and thereby induce antibody-dependent cell-mediated cytotoxicity (ADCC). Furthermore, NK cell activation leads to the production of cytokines, including interferon γ (IFN-γ), macrophage and granulocyte–macrophage colony-stimulating factor (M-CSF, GM-CSF), interleukin-3 (IL-3) and tumour necrosis factor α (TNF-α). These cytokines effect neutrophil recruitment and function, in addition to helping to activate the monocyte/macrophage system. NK cells can lyse virus-infected cells and may be able to lyse tumour cells.

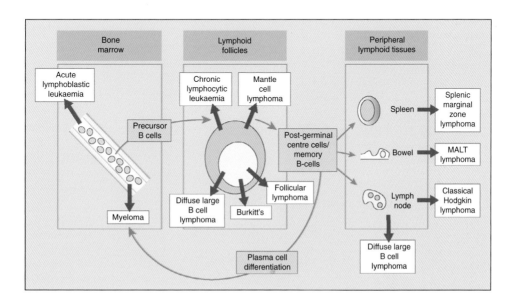

Figure 6.5 Lymphomas arise from 'normal cellular components' of the immune system. Pregerminal centre cells may give rise to CLL or mantle cell lymphoma. The majority of other lymphomas arise from mutations in cells derived from the germinal centre or the postgerminal centre. *Source:* Courtesy of Professor David Mason.

Cellular origin of lymphomas

The vast majority of lymphomas are of B-cell origin; T-cell lymphoma only accounts for approximately 10% of all lymphomas. Lymphomas may arise from any of the stages of T-cell or B-cell maturation. Lymphoma cells have the distinctive morphology and immunophenotype of normal stages of differentiation, which allows them to be classified according to their postulated cell of origin. Figure 6.5 shows how the malignant B-cell disorders relate to the stages of maturation as B cells journey through the lymph nodes and other lymphoid structures.

7

Lymphomas: General principles

Learning objectives

- ✓ To understand the term 'lymphoma' and the difference between Hodgkin lymphoma and non-Hodgkin lymphoma
- ✓ To understand the difference between high- and low-grade lymphoma
- ✓ To be familiar with the principles of staging and to have an awareness of diagnostic techniques used in lymphoma
- ✓ To have a broad understanding of treatment approaches

Lymphomas are *clonal malignant disorders* that derive from *lymphoid cells*, either precursor or mature T cells or B cells. They are divided into two broad categories: *Hodgkin lymphoma* and *non-Hodgkin lymphoma*. Hodgkin lymphoma is diagnosed histologically by the presence of Reed–Sternberg cells (Figure 7.1) within the appropriate cellular background (p. 76).

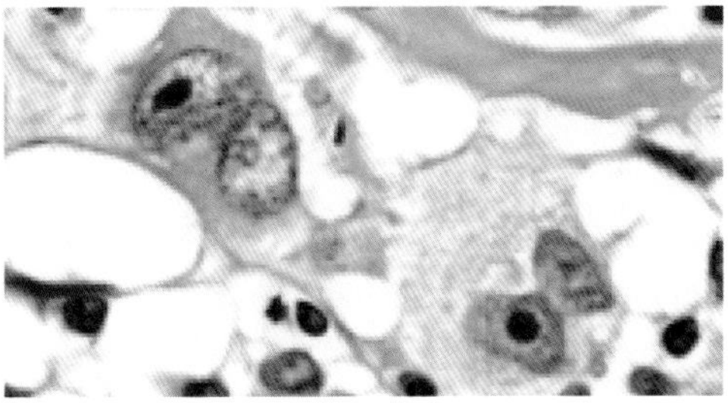

Figure 7.1 Two Reed–Sternberg cells: their presence defines Hodgkin lymphoma.

Lymphomas versus leukaemias

There is often confusion regarding the difference between leukaemias and lymphomas. When classifying malignancies, the important question is always to determine the cell of origin. This is exactly how lymphomas are defined: all arise from lymphocytes or their precursors. However, the term leukaemia is not restricted to any cell of origin: it simply implies the presence of abnormal white cells in the blood. It follows therefore that some conditions (e.g. chronic lymphocytic leukaemia) can fit into both groups. Rather than trying to classify haematological malignancies as leukaemias or lymphomas, it is more logical and much simpler to classify them as lymphoid or myeloid in their origin. By way of example, small lymphocytic lymphoma and chronic lymphocytic leukaemia arise from the same cell of origin; their biology is identical and their treatment is also equivalent. Classifying one as a leukaemia and one as a lymphoma is a biologically irrelevant distinction; classifying both by their cell of origin enhances the understanding of their underlying disease.

Haematology Lecture Notes, Ninth edition. C.S.R. Hatton, N.C. Hughes-Jones, D. Hay and D. Keeling. © 2013 John Wiley & Sons, Ltd.
Published 2013 by John Wiley & Sons, Ltd.

Lymphomas

Aetiology and epidemiology

Lymphomas are more common in males and in older people. Marked variations in racial incidence, histology and immunological subtypes occur around the world. The aetiology of lymphomas is generally unknown, although certain types are associated with specific infectious agents and chronic antigen stimulation. Epstein–Barr virus (EBV) is present in over 90% of cases of endemic Burkitt lymphoma and human T-cell leukaemia virus 1 (HTLV-1) is associated with a very aggressive form of T-cell lymphoma found in Japan and Caribbean countries (ATLL). Some cases of gastric lymphoma are known to be triggered by infection with the bacterium *Helicobacter pylori*. Autoimmune disorders such rheumatoid arthritis and Hashimoto's thyroiditis are associated with a higher incidence of lymphoma.

Cytogenetics and molecular considerations

Cytogenetic analysis has identified a number of specific recurring abnormalities that are associated with certain lymphomas. The alteration of expression of genes involved in cell proliferation, cell differentiation and apoptosis results from these specific genetic alterations.

In 75% of Burkitt lymphomas, translocation of the *c-MYC* gene on chromosome 8 to a site close to the enhancer of the immunoglobulin heavy chain gene locus on chromosome 14 leads to up-regulation and expression of the c-MYC protein, causing cell proliferation and a failure of apoptosis (Figure 7.2). The remaining 25% of Burkitt lymphomas involve translocations of *c-MYC* to the proximity of the genes coding the κ and λ light chains – t(2;8) and t(8;22). Identification of these genetic and molecular abnormalities not only sheds light on the mechanisms of disease, but provides valuable diagnostic information.

Such molecular subclassification allows the identification of lymphomas that have different clinical outcomes with treatment and therefore may help define treatment strategies. They may also identify specific molecular targets for treatment. *Gene expression profiling* (a technique capable of determining the expression of thousands of genes and allowing comparison of the gene expression of one malignant disorder to another using a *microarray*) is helping to identify subsets of lymphomas within the main categories. Diffuse large cell lymphoma is generally thought to be a heterogeneous collection of lymphomas and gene expression studies using microarrays have identified three distinctive patterns of gene expression. Approximately half the patients affected with DLBCL are found to have an activated B-cell phenotype (ABC), whereas the majority of the others have phenotypes that suggest they are derived from the germinal centre (GC type). It is now know that the ABC type has a worse outcome than the GC type (see Figure 7.3).

Clinicians often divide lymphoid disorders into low and high grade (Table 7.1). High-grade lymphomas are those that are rapidly fatal if left untreated but can sometimes be cured with multiagent chemotherapy. Low-grade lymphomas generally have a low proliferation rate and can be controlled with mild chemotherapy, but are incurable (Fig. 7.4).

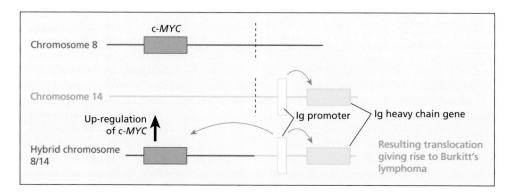

Figure 7.2 Upregulation of c-*MYC* in Burkitt lymphoma. A translocation between chromosome 14 and chromosome 8 juxtaposes the c-*MYC* oncogene with the immunoglobulin heavy chain gene promoter, thereby up-regulating the oncogene c-*MYC* and driving the cell into cycle. The translocation of an oncogene to the vicinity of the Ig gene promoter is a common feature in B-cell lymphomas.

Box 7.1 Gene expression profiling

The division of DLBCL into ABC and GC types was accomplished using gene expression profiling by microarray technology. This technology allows the simultaneous analysis of the expression levels of thousands of genes in cells or tissues of interest.

The study of gene expression by DNA microarray technology is based on the hybridization of messenger RNA (mRNA) to a high-density array of immobilized target sequences, each corresponding to a specific gene. Sample mRNAs are labelled as a complex mixture, usually by incorporation of a fluorescent nucleotide. The labelled pool of sample mRNA is subsequently hybridized to the array, where each messenger will quantitatively hybridize to its complementary sequence. After washing, the fluorescence at each spot on the array is a quantitative measure corresponding to the expression level of the particular gene. The use of two differently labelled mRNA samples allows a quantitative comparison of gene expression in both samples (Figure 7.3). More recently, the technology of RNA sequencing has expanded, with a view to further investigating the gene expression changes in disease: this method uses high throughput next generation sequencing technology to assess the entire transcriptome of a sample, and can detect changes in expression across the whole genome.

Gene expression profiling can be used to compare gene expression in different cell types or tissue types, for example cancer versus normal cells, and to examine changes in gene expression at different stages in the cell cycle or during development. The identification of new target genes and pathways should allow the development of specific molecular-based anticancer drugs. In addition, expression profiles will permit tumour classification into more homogeneous groups and will help identify prognostic groups, as well as the identification of new clinically and biologically relevant tumour entities.

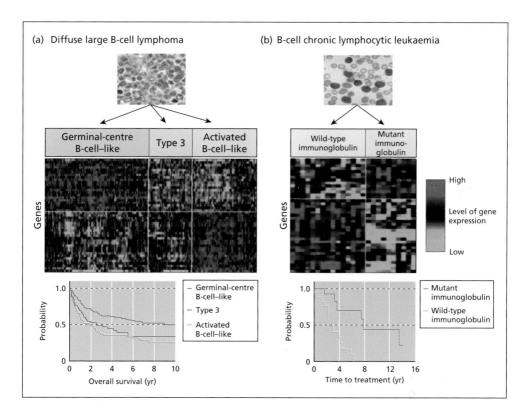

Figure 7.3 cDNA microarray containing 10,000 spots showing differential gene expression. *Notes*: Red – high gene expression; green – low gene expression.

Table 7.1 Examples of high- and low-grade lymphoid neoplasms.

Waldenstrom's macroglobulinaemia	Low grade
Follicular lymphoma	Low grade
Chronic lymphocytic leukaemia	Low grade
Mantle cell lymphoma	Low grade
Diffuse large B-cell lymphoma	High grade
Acute lymphoblastic leukaemia/ lymphoblastic lymphoma	High grade
Burkitt lymphoma	High grade

The division of lymphomas into high or low grade is too imprecise to use as a definitive method for classifying lymphomas or directing treatment. Mantle cell lymphoma is an example of a low-grade lymphoma in terms of its low proliferation rate and incurability, but has the worst prognosis of any lymphoma. Low-grade lymphomas may transform into high-grade tumours that require treatment with combination chemotherapy (Figure 7.5).

Clinical manifestations

Many lymphomas will present as a lump, in which case reaching the diagnosis is generally straightforward. However, some cases may present diagnostic difficulties. Lymphomas are great mimickers of other diseases. They present with weight loss, fever or sweats and are a serious consideration in a patient with pyrexia of unknown origin. Pruritus is another symptom that should offer an alert for the diagnosis of lymphoma. Lymphomas may cause obstruction of the bile duct (nodes in the porta hepatis) or block the renal outflow tract.

Nodal and extranodal lymphomas

About 60% of lymphomas involve the lymph nodes; the remaining 40% may involve almost any organ of the body.

Diagnosis is made by biopsy

The diagnosis is based on the histological appearances of an enlarged lymph node or other affected tissue or the cytology of blood or cerebrospinal fluid (CSF), usually backed up by immunophenotyping and other techniques (outlined below).

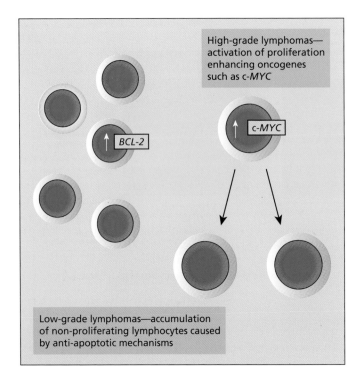

High-grade lymphomas—activation of proliferation enhancing oncogenes such as c-MYC

c-MYC

BCL-2

Low-grade lymphomas—accumulation of non-proliferating lymphocytes caused by anti-apoptotic mechanisms

Figure 7.4 Schematic diagram to illustrate the molecular difference between 'low'- and 'high'-grade lymphomas.

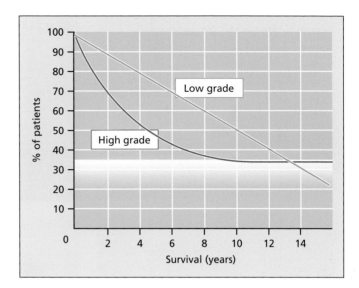

Figure 7.5 Schematic diagram showing outcome for low- and high-grade lymphomas.

Immunophenotyping

The identification of cell-type-specific proteins using labelled antibodies can be very helpful for diagnosis. The process of categorizing the antigenic molecules and epitopes associated with human white cells began in the 1980s. Following a series of workshops, there is now an internationally agreed basis for the nomenclature of leucocyte molecules, the CD scheme.

For example, B cells express an array of different proteins not normally expressed by T cells and other haemopoietic cells. CD20 is one such molecule, almost exclusively expressed on B cells during the middle stage of their development. The anti-CD20 antibody will bind to cells expressing CD20, thereby identifying the cell as being of B-cell origin. The function of CD20 is not fully known. CD19, CD22 and CD79 are other examples of B-cell-expressed molecules identified by antibody binding. The use of labelled antibodies against cells in suspension or on paraffin sections allows identification of expressed antigens (see also the section on flow cytometry' in Chapter 5, Figure 7.6).

Staging

Once the diagnosis of lymphoma has been made by biopsy or examination of blood, pleural fluid or perhaps CSF, staging should be undertaken (Table 7.2). *PET/CT or CT scanning* is the mainstay of staging (Figure 7.7).

Imaging will demonstrate the extent of enlarged lymph nodes, whether the liver and spleen are enlarged and whether other organs are involved. *Bone marrow biopsy* is important in non-Hodgkin lymphoma due to the high frequency of bone marrow involvement in this disorder. Hodgkin lymphoma rarely affects the bone marrow, as its principal mode of spread is lymphatic rather than haematogenous. Measurement of serum lactate dehydrogenase (LDH) is important, as the presence of a raised level is known to confer a poor prognosis in some types of lymphoma. Immunoglobulins should be measured and monoclonal proteins sought by immunoelectrophoresis.

Prognosis

The prognosis of non-Hodgkin lymphoma depends on the clinical entity; that is, whether it is follicular, diffuse large B-cell lymphoma, Burkitt and so on. However, for any of these lymphoma types there are a number of independent prognostic markers, which can be put together to provide a disease specific prognostic index. (Table 7.3 and Figure 7.8).

Treatment and management

A number of different modalities are used in the treatment of lymphoma. Chemotherapy, radiotherapy, antibody treatment and bone marrow transplantation are all used, either alone or in combination. Localized Hodgkin lymphoma and indolent lymphomas can be

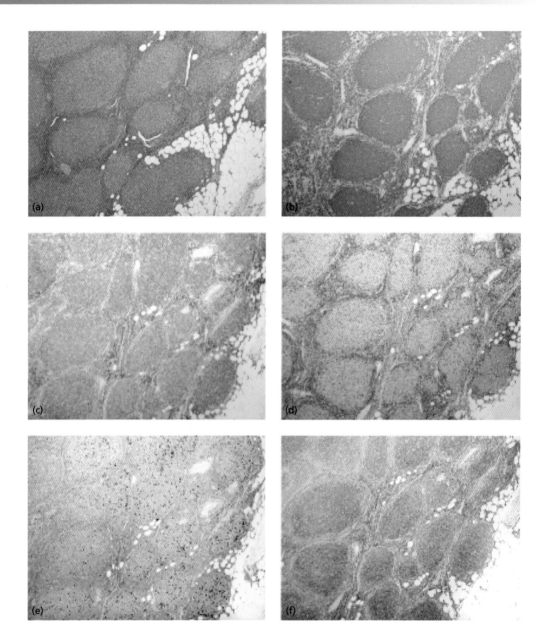

Figure 7.6 Typical immunophenotype of follicular lymphoma (paraffin section): (a) H&E, (b) CD20, (c) bcl-2, (d) CD3, (e) Ki67 and (f) CD10. *Source*: Courtesy of Professor Kevin Gatter.

Table 7.2 **Staging of lymphomas.**

Stage I	Involvement of a single lymph node group
Stage II	Involvement of two or more lymph node groups on one side of the diaphragm
Stage III	Involvement of lymph node groups on both sides of the diaphragm
Stage IV	Involvement of extralymphatic sites (e.g. bone marrow or liver)

Note: Patients are said to be symptom stage (A) if they have no systemic symptoms, or symptom stage (B) in the presence of any one of night sweats, fever or weight loss (10% loss in past six months).

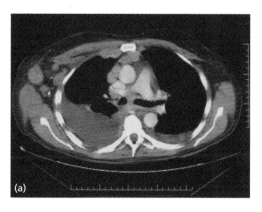 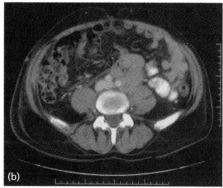

Figure 7.7 CT image of a lymphoma: (a) right axillary, anterior mediastinal nodal disease and bilateral pleural effusions; and (b) bulky retroperitoneal lymphadenopathy (i.v. and bowel contrast help define the lymphomatous masses).

Table 7.3 The international prognostic index: Features conferring a worse prognosis in patients with diffuse large B-cell lymphoma.

Presence of extranodal disease: Disease outside lymphatic sites confers a poor prognosis

Advanced stage disease: Worse prognosis

Elevated LDH: Worse prognosis

Performance status: Patients who are unable to care for themselves or are confined to bed have a worse prognosis

Age: Increasing age is associated with a poor prognosis

very effectively treated by radiotherapy. Widespread lymphomas require chemotherapy, either single or multiagent. Recently, a number of different antibodies against leucocyte-specific molecules have been developed for therapy. One such antibody (rituximab) targets CD20 and has been found to have good activity in follicular and other lymphomas expressing this molecule (Figure 7.9). Coupling these antibodies to radioactive isotopes appears to lead to improved response rates (e.g. ^{90}Y-labelled anti-CD20 antibodies). Restaging during treatment may guide the number of courses of chemotherapy. Staging PET/CT scans are usually performed at the end of treatment to document the response: either complete remission (CR), partial remission (PR) >50% reduction in the size of the mass, stable disease (SD) or progressive disease (PD).

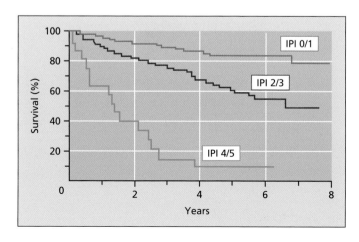

Figure 7.8 The overall survival of patients with follicular lymphoma subdivided by the IPI score $p < 0.001$ for differences between the curves.

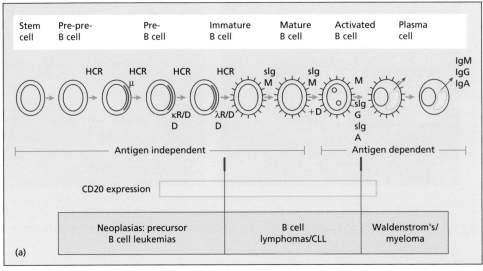

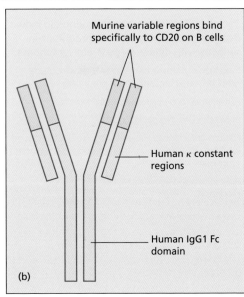

Figure 7.9 (a) The diagram shows the changes that occur during the maturation of a stem cell into plasma cells. Note that immature B cells and plasma cells do not express CD20. *Notes:* CLL – chronic lymphocytic leukaemia; HCR – heavy chain rearrangement; μ – mu heavy chain synthesis; κR/D – kappa chain rearrangement or deletion; λR/D – lambda chain rearrangement or deletion; sIgM, sIgG, sIgA – surface immunoglobulins M, G and A, respectively. (b) A schematic diagram of rituximab, a chimeric monoclonal antibody designed to bind to CD20 antigen on B cells inducing apoptosis and cell death.

8

Classification of lymphoma

Learning objectives

✓ To understand the basis for the classification of lymphoma
✓ To appreciate that lymphoma is first divided into Hodgkin and non-Hodgkin subtypes
✓ To understand that the cell of origin is important in classification

Classification of lymphomas has been perceived as being complex and difficult. The WHO 2001 classification (Table 8.1) aims to classify lymphomas according to morphological, genetic, molecular, immunophenotypic and clinical features into specific entities. The classification uses the cell of origin as its basis – T, B or NK cells. The lymphomas are divided into those that are derived from precursor lymphoid cells and those derived from more mature cells (Tables 8.2 and 8.3; Figures 8.1 and 8.2). Hodgkin lymphoma is defined by the presence of the Reed–Sternberg cell and is divided into two types, classical Hodgkin lymphoma and lymphocyte-predominant Hodgkin Lymphoma.

Unlike many of the former classifications, the WHO classification is useful to clinicians because it recognizes distinct lymphoma entities that may require specific treatment and management programmes. It is likely that within the current classification there will be additional entities not yet identified, which will be realized through a combination of immunophenotyping, cytogenetics and molecular analysis. The ability to look at differential gene expression profiles may be helpful in this respect.

Table 8.1 Hodgkin lymphomas.

Classical	
Nodular sclerosing	The commonest type in young patients
Mixed cellularity	Second most common, may have worse prognosis
Lymphocyte deplete	
Lymphocyte rich	
Non-classical	
Lymphocyte predominant	Behaves more like a low-grade non-Hodgkin lymphoma

Haematology Lecture Notes, Ninth edition. C.S.R. Hatton, N.C. Hughes-Jones, D. Hay and D. Keeling. © 2013 John Wiley & Sons, Ltd.
Published 2013 by John Wiley & Sons, Ltd.

Table 8.2 Non-Hodgkin B-cell lymphomas.

Precursor B-cell neoplasms

Precursor B-lymphoblastic leukaemia/lymphoma (ALL)	ALL is the commonest type of leukaemia found in children. Fatal if left untreated; needs multiagent chemotherapy with prophylactic CNS treatment to prevent CNS relapse

Peripheral B-cell neoplasms

B-cell chronic lymphocytic leukaemia/small lymphocytic lymphoma (CLL/SLL)	CLL is the commonest type of leukaemia found in adults over 50 years. Presents with lymphocytosis, progresses to lymphadenopathy, hepatosplenomegaly and bone marrow failure. Treatment is usually with oral chemotherapy
Lymphoplasmacytic/ Waldenstrom's macroglobulinaemia (WM)	Indolent lymphoma presenting with bone marrow involvement, lymphadenopathy and hepatosplenomegaly. Typically has IgM paraprotein, which may cause hyperviscosity or coagulation problems (WM type)
Mantle cell lymphoma (MCL)	MCL presents with widespread lymphadenopathy, hepatosplenomegaly, bone marrow and extranodal (especially GI tract) involvement. Very poor prognosis
Follicular lymphoma (FL)	Indolent lymphoma presenting with lymphadenopathy, bone marrow involvement and hepatosplenomegaly. 30% rate of transformation to large-cell lymphoma. Treatment with a combination of chemotherapy plus rituximab imparts the best outcome. Maintenance rituximab recently shown to be of benefit
Marginal zone B-cell lymphoma (includes MALT lymphomas and splenic lymphoma)	Usually extranodal lymphomas. The commonest mucosa-associated lymphoma affects the stomach. Often associated with *Helicobacter pylori* infection. May be widespread
Hairy cell leukaemia (HCL)	Presents with pancytopenia, circulating hairy cells and splenomegaly. Treatment with chemotherapy leads to sustained remissions
Plasmacytoma/myeloma	See Chapter 10
Diffuse large B-cell lymphoma (DLBCL)	Aggressive and common lymphoma. Frequently presents with weight loss, fever, sweats and lymphadenopathy. Good response rates to a combination of rituximab and CHOP chemotherapy. Curable in >50% of cases
Burkitt lymphoma (BL)	Highly aggressive. Frequent extranodal involvement. Needs sequential multiagent chemotherapy

Table 8.3 Non-Hodgkin T-cell lymphomas.

Precursor T-cell neoplasm

Precursor T-lymphoblastic leukaemia/ lymphoma	T cell ALL – for clinical picture, see B cell ALL above

Peripheral T-cell and NK-cell neoplasms

T-cell prolymphocytic leukaemia	Rare, aggressive leukaemia responds poorly to chemotherapy. Better response rates to antibody therapy – Alemtuzumab
Large granular lymphocyte leukaemia (LGL)	Rare CD8+ve indolent lymphoma associated with neutropenia
Mycosis fungoides, Sezary syndrome	Rare CD4+ve lymphomas affecting the skin. MF is often indolent in the early stages
Peripheral T-cell lymphomas, unspecified (PTC)	Widespread nodal disease associated with systemic symptoms – progress despite chemotherapy
Angioimmunoblastic T-cell lymphoma (AILD)	Rare aggressive lymphoma associated with fever, lymphadenopathy, skin rashes and Coombs positive haemolytic anaemia. Poor prognosis
Enteropathy-associated T-cell lymphoma (EATL)	Aggressive lymphoma associated with adult-onset coeliac disease
Adult T-cell lymphoma/leukaemia (ATL/L)	HTLV-1-associated lymphoma found with high prevalence in Japan, Caribbean and south-eastern USA. Usually very aggressive clinical course, often complicated by hypercalcaemia. Many patients relapse in the CNS
Anaplastic large-cell lymphoma (ALCL)	Occurs in childhood and young adults. Aggressive, but many cases do well with combination chemotherapy

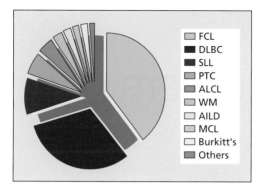

Figure 8.1 Pie chart showing the relative incidence of different non-Hodgkin lymphomas. For abbreviations see Tables 8.2 and 8.3.

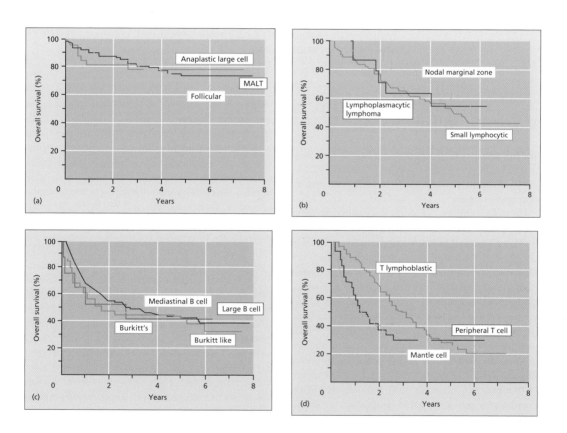

Figure 8.2 Survival curves for patients with different types of lymphoma. (a, b) Good prognosis lymphomas. (c, d) Poor prognosis lymphomas (note that mantle cell lymphoma (MCL) has the worst prognosis of any lymphoma).

9

Neoplastic disorders of lymphoid cells

Learning objectives

✓ To know the pathological changes, clinical presentation, investigation and principles of management of Hodgkin lymphoma
✓ To know the pathological changes, clinical manifestations and the basic principles of treatment of the commoner non-Hodgkin lymphomas, including acute lymphoblastic leukaemia (ALL), chronic lymphocytic leukaemia (CLL), diffuse large B-cell lymphoma (DLBCL) and follicular lymphoma (FL).

Hodgkin lymphoma

The first description of this disorder has been accredited to Dr Thomas Hodgkin of Guy's Hospital, following his account in 1832 of affected lymph glands in postmortem cases.

Hodgkin lymphoma is one of the commoner lymphomas seen in Western countries and is characterized by the presence of a low number of tumour cells, designated Hodgkin's/Reed–Sternberg cells. The Reed–Sternberg cells are bi- or multinucleate, with each nucleus containing one prominent nucleolus. Other Hodgkin's cells are mononucleate. The histological findings in a lymph node affected by Hodgkin lymphoma are scattered tumour cells admixed with reactive lymphocytes, plasma cells, macrophages, neutrophils, eosinophils and a variable amount of fibrosis. Under the term 'Hodgkin lymphoma' are recognized two clinically and biologically different entities: classic Hodgkin lymphoma, of which there are four histological types (Table 9.1); and non-classic Hodgkin lymphoma, which includes the entity of lymphocyte-predominant Hodgkin lymphoma (LPHL). Nodular sclerosis is the commonest histological subtype and is characterized by bands of fibrosis that enclose nodules of lymphoid tissue containing variable numbers of Hodgkin's cells (Figure 9.1). Mixed cellularity Hodgkin lymphoma is characterized by the presence of a heterogeneous mixture of lymphocytes, eosinophils, neutrophils, plasma cells, epithelial cells and Hodgkin's cells. In general, the more lymphocytes present, the fewer the number of Hodgkin's cells and the better the prognosis. Lymphocyte-depleted Hodgkin lymphoma is a rare form and is characterized by a low number of lymphocytes, by the absence of fibrous bands and by numerous, sometimes anaplastic, Hodgkin's/Reed–Sternberg cells. LPHL has a chronic relapsing course and often behaves more like follicular non-Hodgkin lymphoma (see below).

Whereas the B-cell nature of the tumour cells (called 'popcorn' cells or lymphocytic and histiocytic cells) of LPHL has been widely accepted, the cellular origin of the Reed–Sternberg cells of classic Hodgkin lymphoma has been the subject of debate for many years. This was due to fact that although Reed–Sternberg cells express the lymphocyte-associated marker CD30, they do not consistently stain with markers for B or T cells. However, molecular techniques using single Reed–Sternberg cells microdissected from tissue sections have demonstrated that cells harbour clonal immunoglobulin

Haematology Lecture Notes, Ninth edition. C.S.R. Hatton, N.C. Hughes-Jones, D. Hay and D. Keeling. © 2013 John Wiley & Sons, Ltd.
Published 2013 by John Wiley & Sons, Ltd.

Table 9.1 Rye classification of the histological appearances of lymph nodes in classical Hodgkin lymphoma.

Subgroup	Characteristics	Cases (%)	Surviving 5 years (%)
Lymphocyte rich	Infiltrate consists largely of small lymphocytes. There are only a few eosinophils, Reed–Sternberg cells and mononuclear Hodgkin's cells	15	70
Nodular sclerosing	The node is divided by broad bands of connective tissue into nodules containing a mixture of Reed–Sternberg cells, mononuclear Hodgkin's cells, lymphocytes, plasma cells, macrophages and eosinophils	40	60
Mixed cellularity	There are no broad bands of connective tissue. The node is diffusely infiltrated with the same mixture of cell types as above. Reed–Sternberg cells are readily seen. Fibrosis and focal necrosis are common	30	30
Lymphocyte depleted	Mononuclear Hodgkin's cells and Reed–Sternberg cells are present in large numbers. Relatively few lymphocytes are seen and there may be diffuse fibrosis	15	20

gene rearrangements, thereby demonstrating Reed–Sternberg cells to be of B-cell origin.

Incidence and aetiology

Whereas the incidence of non-Hodgkin lymphoma increased in the 1980s and 1990s, the incidence of Hodgkin lymphoma has remained stable at about

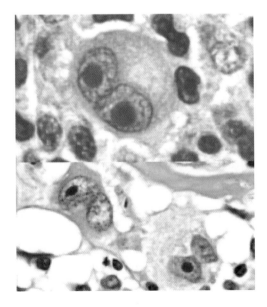

Figure 9.1 Photomicrograph showing Reed–Sternberg cells from a case of Hodgkin lymphoma.

3 per 100,000 population; it is higher in men than in women. Hodgkin lymphoma increases in incidence with age, peaking in the third decade, followed by a decline. It used to be thought that there was a second peak in later life, but this has not been verified in recent studies. The nodular sclerosis type tends to occur in young adults.

The aetiology of Hodgkin lymphoma is unknown. The apparent geographical clustering of cases that has been reported has suggested an infectious aetiology and many efforts have been made to identify likely culprits. However, it seems that such clustering may have occurred by chance alone. Epstein–Barr virus (EBV) has long remained a favoured possible cause, because similar age groups are affected by both Hodgkin lymphoma and glandular fever. Indeed, there is some evidence that EBV might have a part to play in the aetiology of Hodgkin lymphoma, supported by the finding of clonal EBV DNA in 30–40% of cases.

Clinical features

The clinical features resemble those found in non-Hodgkin lymphoma. Lymph node enlargement is the commonest presentation, usually affecting the neck and mediastinum (Figure 9.2). Spread is mainly along the lymph vessels; hence lymph node involvement tends to be contiguous. Sweats, fever, weight loss and pruritus may occur. Alcohol-induced pain in affected lymph nodes is thought to be virtually diagnostic. A not-infrequent presentation of Hodgkin lymphoma in young patients is cough, chest pain or dyspnoea as

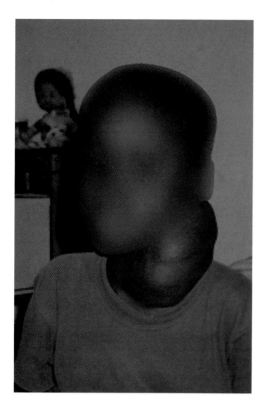

Figure 9.2 Massive cervical lymphadenopathy in a young boy with Hodgkin lymphoma.

a result of extensive intrathoracic disease. Diagnosis is made by lymph node biopsy. The staging system using CT scanning is the same as that used for non-Hodgkin lymphoma (Table 9.2), except that the bone marrow is very rarely involved. A full blood count, erythrocyte sedimentation rate (ESR), liver function

Table 9.2 Basic features of the Ann Arbor staging system.

Stages	Characteristics
I	Involvement of one lymph node area
II	Involvement of two or more lymph node areas on the same side of the diaphragm
III	Involvement of lymph nodes on both sides of the diaphragm with or without involvement of the spleen
IV	Involvement of one or more extranodal sites (e.g. liver, marrow, lung)

Notes: A – without systemic symptoms; B – with systemic symptoms (night sweats, fever, weight loss).

tests, renal and bone profile and lactate dehydrogenase (LDH) are all necessary and may confer prognostic information.

Prognosis

A number of attempts have been made to predict outcome in patients treated for Hodgkin lymphoma. The prognosis is worse for males, older patients, patients with advanced disease and those with a low serum albumin concentration, anaemia and leucocytosis. Understanding prognostic factors may enable more intensive treatment to be given to patients with a predicted worse outcome, while those patients with a good prognosis could be spared unnecessary toxicity and adverse late effects.

Treatment

The goal of treatment for Hodgkin lymphoma is cure, while minimizing complications. Early-stage disease (stages IA–IIA) can be effectively treated with abbreviated chemotherapy together with localized radiotherapy. Patients who relapse can often be salvaged using combination chemotherapy or high-dose chemotherapy with peripheral blood stem-cell rescue.

Advanced disease (stages IIB–IV) is treated with six to eight courses of combination chemotherapy; radiotherapy is reserved to treat residual masses or given after completion of chemotherapy to areas previously involved by bulky disease. Modern treatment is based on a number of considerations, most notably the need to attain a high cure rate, the need to minimize the toxicity of treatment and the need to preserve fertility. The high 'cure' rate in Hodgkin lymphoma may be at the price of a higher death rate from second malignancies and other toxicities. Use of alkylating agents and radiotherapy is likely to contribute to this excess risk. This increase in death rate from 'non-Hodgkin' causes is graphically illustrated in Figure 9.3. After 15 years from the diagnosis, the mortality from causes other than Hodgkin lymphoma is greater than deaths due to the lymphoma itself, although this trend may change as patients are treated with modern chemotherapy regimens that aim to reduce long-term toxicity. Irradiation of peripubertal breast tissue is thought to put patients at particularly high risk of breast cancer.

While early-stage Hodgkin lymphoma can be cured with radiotherapy, it was not until cyclical four-drug chemotherapy regimens such as MOPP were used in the late 1960s that advanced-stage disease could be cured. MOPP (*mustine*

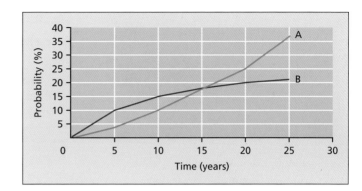

Figure 9.3 Actuarial risk of death from Hodgkin lymphoma (B) or other causes (A) in patients treated for Hodgkin lymphoma.

(alkylating agent), vincristine (*Oncovin*), prednisolone and *procarbazine*), although very effective in at least half of all cases, has been found to be associated with secondary leukaemia (myelodysplasia and acute myeloblastic leukaemia) and a high incidence of infertility. Regimens containing Doxorubicin (Adriamycin; e.g. ABVD: Adriamycin, Bleomycin, Vinblastine, Dacarbazine) are favoured for initial treatment because of the low incidence of secondary leukaemia and the fact that most patients, both male and female, remain fertile. ABVD has been shown to be equally effective to MOPP-like regimens. ABVD is myelosuppressive and two drugs of this four-drug regimen are associated with serious side effects: the use of bleomycin can cause significant pulmonary toxicity and exposure to high doses of anthracyclines is known to cause cardiomyopathy. The latter two problems can be avoided by close monitoring and discontinuation of the drug that is responsible.

Patients who fail to respond to initial therapy, or who relapse, can be considered for high-dose therapy with peripheral blood stem-cell rescue. Approximately 40% of such patients respond well to this approach (see Chapter 12).

Positron emission tomography scanning

Positron emission tomography (*PET scanning*) may be useful to determine whether there is active disease in residual masses after the completion of therapy. The uptake of a radioactive fluorinated glucose molecule in active tumours may dictate whether further treatment such as radiotherapy is necessary. Recent evidence suggests that PET negativity following therapy carries a much improved prognosis when cases are compared with those that are PET positive.

Non-Hodgkin lymphomas

Acute lymphoblastic leukaemia (ALL)

Pathology

Precursor lymphoblastic neoplasms of B-cell or T-cell type usually present as a leukaemia with circulating blast cells (acute lymphoblastic leukaemia, ALL); however, they may also present as a mediastinal mass with few circulating blast cells (the lymphoblastic lymphomas). In the leukaemic form, the marrow is heavily infiltrated with blast cells, which are also present in the peripheral blood (Figure 9.4).

The disorder results from a clonal proliferation of cells from the earliest stages of lymphoid maturation (i.e. B or T blast cells). B-cell leukaemia blast cells have a phenotype defined by the presence of CD19, CD79a, CD10, CD34 and terminal deoxynucleotidyl transferase (TdT). T-cell markers such as CD7 and CD3 will define the cells as being of T-cell origin.

Cytogenetics

Cytogenetic analysis provides important prognostic information. Treatment regimens are increasingly based on risk stratification and therefore cytogenetics is an important part of the investigations at presentation. Hyperdiploidy (increased numbers of chromosomes beyond the diploid state) generally carries a good prognosis, whereas certain structural variants such as the presence of a Philadelphia chromosome t(9;22) are found in about 5% of children with ALL and this confers a very poor prognosis. Other poor prognostic findings include rearrangements of the *MLL* (mixed lineage leukaemia/lymphoma) gene and hypodiploidy.

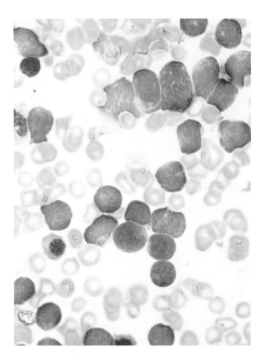

Figure 9.4 Bone marrow smear from a case of ALL. The blasts are small or medium-sized and have scanty cytoplasm. The nuclei have fine but densely packed, homogeneous-appearing chromatin and the nucleoli are small.

Clinical and laboratory features

ALL is the commonest childhood cancer, but may present at any age. In children, the peak incidence is between the ages of 2 and 4 years. The clinical manifestations are listed in Box 9.1, as are the laboratory findings. Most of the clinical manifestations can be explained in terms of bone marrow failure secondary to bone marrow infiltration.

Treatment

Treatment of childhood acute leukaemia has improved greatly, due largely to the results of clinical trials that have been conducted over the last 20–30 years. Risk stratification based on prognostic factors including minimal residual disease is used to determine the protocols on which children and adults with ALL are treated, though the general schema is outlined below. The treatment is by chemotherapy, given in four phases:

1   *Induction*: The aim of induction chemotherapy is to clear the bone marrow of leukaemia blast cells and replace them with normal haemopoietic cells.

Box 9.1

Clinical features of ALL

Symptoms and their pathological basis
- Weakness, tiredness, malaise, lassitude
- Bruising and bleeding secondary to thrombocytopenia
- Otitis media, pharyngitis, pneumonia or fever due to bacterial infection caused by profound neutropenia
- Bone pain
- Enlarged lymph nodes
- Headache and vomiting resulting from CNS involvement leading to increased intracranial pressure

Physical findings
- Pallor
- Petechial haemorrhages, purpura and bruising
- Lymphadenopathy
- Hepatosplenomegaly
- Bone tenderness
- Fever

Laboratory features of ALL
- Anaemia
- Leucopenia
- Thrombocytopenia
- Blood film may show circulating blast cells
- Bone marrow usually heavily infiltrated with blast cells (>20%)

---

2   *Consolidation*: Consolidation therapy reduces the leukaemia cell burden further and uses a combination of moderately intensive treatment after normal haemopoiesis has been restored with induction chemotherapy.

3   *CNS prophylaxis*: A phase of prophylactic treatment to prevent central nervous system involvement is always given. This can be achieved by the administration of high-dose chemotherapy drugs such as methotrexate, which cross the blood–brain barrier, or by direct administration of drugs into the cerebrospinal fluid (intrathecal), or by giving external beam radiotherapy.

4   *Maintenance therapy*: The final treatment phase is that of maintenance therapy. Continuous oral and intermittent intravenous chemotherapy is given over 2–3 years.

Prognosis

A number of prognostic factors determine outcome in ALL. Boys do worse than girls and a high white cell count at presentation and an age over 10 years also confer a poor prognosis. Low-risk childhood ALL can be cured in a high percentage of cases. Patients who relapse or who present in the poorest-risk categories should be considered for allogeneic bone marrow transplantation (Chapter 12). Adults with ALL do not have such a good prognosis and may be offered allogeneic bone marrow transplantation in the first remission.

Lymphoblastic lymphoma

This represents the lymphomatous equivalent of ALL (i.e. there is little peripheral blood or bone marrow involvement). It has very similar features to ALL but there are a number of characteristic clinical features: it is commoner in adolescent males and it frequently presents with a mediastinal mass. Patients must have less than 20% blasts in their bone marrow, otherwise they are classified as having ALL. Lymphoblastic lymphoma is treated using the same protocols as for ALL.

B-cell chronic lymphocytic leukaemia

Chronic lymphocytic leukaemia (CLL) is a neoplastic disorder characterized by the accumulation of small mature lymphocytes in the blood (Figure 9.5), bone marrow and lymphoid tissues. This is the commonest leukaemia seen in the Western world and tends to affect almost exclusively adults over the age of 50 years. The disorder is much less common in China, Japan and south-east Asia. The cells that give rise to the disorder express the B-cell markers CD19 and CD20. They also express CD23, are negative for CD10, but express the T-cell marker CD5 and weakly express surface IgM. Cytogenetic studies confer some prognostic information: for example, deletions involving chromosome 17 (p53 deletions) confer a very poor prognosis. The clinical and laboratory features of CLL are summarized in Box 9.2.

Autoimmune phenomena may occur in patients with CLL. The most common manifestations are autoimmune haemolytic anaemia (AIHA) and autoimmune thrombocytopenic purpura (ITP). Patients may rarely develop pure red cell aplasia or neutropenia.

> **Box 9.2**
>
> ### Clinical features of CLL
>
> *Symptoms and their pathological basis*
> - Most patients are over 60 years of age
> - Many patients are asymptomatic at diagnosis
> - Patients may present with symptoms attributable to anaemia – tiredness and fatigue
> - Bruising and bleeding secondary to thrombocytopenia
> - Sinusitis, bacterial pneumonia, secondary to hypogammaglobulinaemia
> - Night sweats, fever and weight loss are uncommon but may occur
>
> ***Physical findings***
> - Lymphadenopathy
> - Hepatosplenomegaly
>
> ### Laboratory features of CLL
> - Monoclonal lymphocytosis is greater than 5×10^9/L
> - In the more advanced stages of the disease there may be anaemia and thrombocytopenia
> - The direct antiglobulin (Coombs) test may be positive
> - Bone marrow aspirate and trephine biopsy demonstrate the extent of bone marrow infiltration
> - Hypogammaglobulinaemia is a common finding – a small proportion of patients will have a monoclonal band on immunoelectrophoresis
> - Immunophenotyping of the malignant lymphocytes shows expression of CD5, CD19, CD20, CD23 and CD79a and surface IgM (weakly positive); CD10 is negative

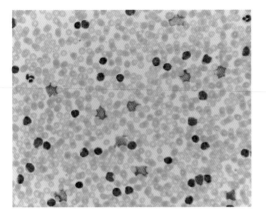

Figure 9.5 Blood film in a patient with B-cell CLL. Note the presence of increased numbers of small lymphocytes and some smear cells.

Acquired angioneurotic oedema may also result from autoimmune antibodies against the C1 esterase inhibitor. The antibodies are not thought to be produced by the malignant B cells, but rather by bystander populations of normal B cells.

CLL has a predictable natural history. Most patients have only a lymphocytosis at the beginning of their illness and progress to develop lymphadenopathy, hepatosplenomegaly and finally bone marrow failure. It is the presence or absence of these features that determines the prognosis. In about 3% of CLL cases, transformation to a large cell lymphoma may occur. Richter's transformation, named after Maurice Richter who originally described this entity in 1928, carries a poor prognosis.

Hypogammaglobulinaemia

Patients with CLL commonly have an associated hypogammaglobulinaemia. Reductions in the serum levels of IgM, IgG and IgA may all occur and these predispose to infections, particularly of the respiratory tract, by capsulated organisms such as *Steptococcus pneumoniae* and *Haemophilus influenzae*. Replacement therapy with intravenous pooled human immunoglobulin can reduce the frequency of respiratory tract infections in such patients.

Small lymphocytic B-cell lymphoma

Small lymphocytic lymphoma (SLL) is the lymphomatous equivalent of CLL without abnormal cells in the peripheral blood, and has the same biology and clinical features. The disease is characterized by lymph node involvement and bone marrow infiltration.

Treatment of CLL/SLL

Patients with CLL/SLL who are asymptomatic often do not require treatment; simple monitoring in the clinic is sufficient. Indications for treatment include systemic symptoms such as sweats, fever, weight loss or cytopenias such as anaemia. Many frail, usually older patients with progressive disease can be safely treated with a simple regimen of oral chlorambucil or, more recently, bendamustine. For younger, fit patients, fludarabine in combination with cyclophosphamide together with rituximab is the treatment of choice (Flu/Cy-R). This combination therapy results in very high response rates (80%), with an average time to progression of approximately three years. Patients with chromosome 17p deletions are refractory to chemotherapy and have a dismal prognosis. Such patients are best treated with a combination of steroids plus alemtuzumab (Campath-1H). Campath is an antibody that targets CD52, an antigen expressed on B and T cells; it has been shown to have activity in CLL, but appears to have particular value in treating cases where p53 on chromosome 17p is deleted. The median survival of all patients with B-cell CLL is 10–12 years. More intensive treatment including bone marrow transplantation is sometimes attempted in younger patients with poor prognostic disease.

Lymphoplasmacytic lymphoma/Waldenström's macroglobulinaemia

This disorder usually behaves in a low-grade fashion. Like CLL, this is a disease found in patients who are in their sixth or seventh decade. The malignant cells are mature B cells capable of secreting IgM. The bone marrow is typically involved, as are the liver and spleen. Lymphadenopathy is also a common feature. The disorder can be dominated by clinical manifestations consequent on high levels of monoclonal IgM; the condition is then known as Waldenström's macroglobulinaemia.

High concentrations of IgM and the accompanying hyperviscosity cause headaches, visual disturbances (fundoscopic examination may reveal dilated veins, papilloedema and retinal haemorrhage) and altered consciousness. There may also be bleeding or thrombosis.

The IgM paraprotein may have unusual physical properties such as causing red cell agglutination (cold agglutinins) or precipitating in cold temperatures (cryoglobulin).

Patients are frequently anaemic and experience symptoms of tiredness and fatigue. The fatigue is often out of proportion to the level of haemoglobin. Systemic symptoms such as fever, weight loss and night sweats may occur, particularly if the lymphoma undergoes high-grade transformation.

Laboratory findings are summarized in Table 9.3.

Table 9.3 Laboratory findings in Waldenström's macroglobulinaemia.
Anaemia
Leucopenia
Thrombocytopenia
Lymphocytosis may occur
IgM monoclonal protein
Bone marrow infiltration with lymphoid cells

Treatment

A combination of an alkylating agent such as cyclophosphamide and prednisolone together with the monoclonal antibody rituximab is a favoured first-line therapy. Patients who fail to respond or later progress can be treated with a fludarabine-containing regimen or the more aggressive R-CHOP combination used to treat large-cell lymphoma. Combination chemotherapy such as CHOP can be useful, particularly if there is high-grade transformation, which occurs in a small percentage of cases. Hyperviscosity syndrome requires urgent plasma exchange.

The immunophenotype is CD20+ve, CD19+ve, CD5-ve, sIg+ve and CD10-ve.

Follicular lymphoma (FL)

Follicular lymphoma is relatively easy for the pathologist to identify because of its follicular growth pattern (see Figure 7.6). The disorder typifies the so-called low-grade lymphomas, being indolent in its clinical course but remaining incurable. Follicular lymphoma is associated with a translocation between chromosome 14 and 18, t(14;18), which leads to the up-regulation of the anti-apoptotic protein BCL-2. The t(14;18) BCL-2 positive B cells are thought to arise in early B cells, which then move into the germinal centre of the lymph node follicle where they acquire additional mutations, causing FL. The presence of the t(14;18) translocation is insufficient to cause follicular lymphoma on its own. In a proportion of cases further additional mutations may cause the lymphoma to transform to a DLBCL type, so-called high grade transformation.

FL is one of the commonest types of lymphoma. Most patients present with widespread lymphadenopathy, bone marrow infiltration and hepatosplenomegaly. Occasionally this lymphoma may present in an extranodal fashion, the gastrointestinal tract and the skin being among the more unusual sites of involvement.

The clinical course alternates between stable periods when patients remain well and periods of progressive disease requiring therapy. High-grade transformation in which there is development of large-cell lymphoma (see below) occurs in 30% of patients and confers a poor prognosis.

There is no evidence that early or intensive treatment of follicular lymphoma at presentation improves outcome. Therapy is required, however, in patients with systemic symptoms, critical organ failure or bulky disease. Randomized controlled trials have shown a survival advantage for the addition of the anti-CD20 antibody rituximab (R) to commonly used first-line chemotherapy regimens such as cyclophosphamide, vincristine and prednisolone (CVP). Patients who relapse after first-line chemotherapy can often be effectively treated with regimens such as R-CHOP or regimens containing fludarabine. Furthermore, there is evidence that maintenance rituximab (given every two or three months over a period of two years) benefits patients who have achieved at least a partial response to either first- or second-line therapy by roughly doubling the time to progression. Patients who respond well to second-line treatment and who are otherwise fit can be considered for more intensive, perhaps even curative, strategies such as high-dose therapy and stem-cell rescue or reduced-intensity conditioning (RIC) allografting. Frail, usually older patients can be treated with the single oral alkylating agent chlorambucil, with or without rituximab.

Low-grade lymphomas are often extremely radiosensitive and radiotherapy can be useful for treating localized or bulky disease. An alternative approach involves conjugating a β-emitting radioisotope to an anti-CD20 antibody. This allows the delivery of radiation directly to the site of disease. This strategy has been shown to be an effective therapy for patients with follicular lymphoma and may be incorporated into future treatment strategies. In addition, other radioisotopes, including γ-emitters, have been linked with anti-CD20 antibodies with the same aim.

The prognosis of follicular lymphoma is variable and is anything from 2 to 20 years. The median survival is about 10–12 years from diagnosis.

The immunophenotype is CD19+ve, CD20+ve, CD10+ve, BCL-2+ve and BCL-6+ve.

Mantle cell lymphoma

Mantle cell lymphoma is an aggressive low-grade lymphoma. This lymphoma entity is commoner in males and generally presents in older patients with a median age of 60 years. The malignant cells are thought to derive from cells of the mantle zone of the lymph node follicle (Figure 9.6(a)). The lymphoma cells are small to medium-sized and in common with CLL express CD5. In contrast to CLL, mantle cell lymphoma does not express CD23 and there is a characteristic cytogenetic abnormality that is found in nearly all cases. A translocation between chromosome 11 and chromosome 14, t(11;14), leads to the up-regulation of the protein cyclin D1, which is known to play a key role in cell-cycle regulation (Figure 9.6(b)).

The disorder presents with widespread lymphadenopathy, hepatosplenomegaly and bone marrow

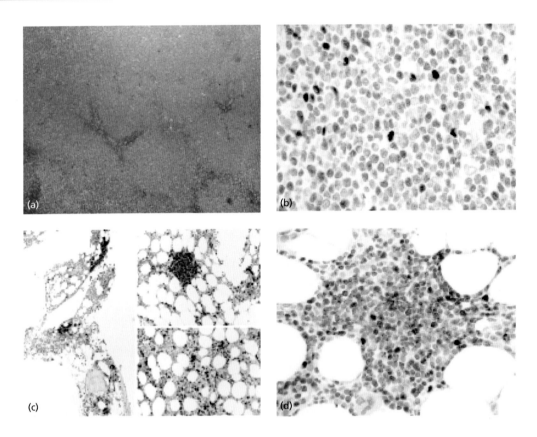

Figure 9.6 (a) The non-specific histological appearance seen in the biopsy of a patient with mantle cell lymphoma; (b) staining using an antibody against cyclin D1, which is overexpressed in mantle cell lymphoma; (c) minimal disease after treatment identified by cyclin D1 staining; and (d) high-power view.

involvement and often abnormal lymphocytes can be seen in the peripheral blood. Some series have reported a very high incidence of gastrointestinal involvement (80%). Systemic symptoms are unusual, most patients feeling reasonably well at the time of presentation. The disease runs an aggressive course, with a mean survival of 2–4 years. The disorder is not curable and, although intensive chemotherapy is often given, there is no very effective therapy. For younger, fit patients with aggressive disease who have responded to chemotherapy, high-dose therapy or RIC allograft should be considered.

The immunophenotype is CD19+ve, CD20+ve, CD5+ve, CD23+ve, IgM+ve and cyclin D1+ve.

Hairy cell leukaemia

This uncommon disorder frequently affects middle-aged males. It typically presents with pancytopenia and splenomegaly. Characteristic hairy cells are usually found on examination of a peripheral blood film (Figure 9.7). The disorder is diagnosed by microscopy of the blood and bone marrow examination. Immunophenotyping and cytochemistry help to define the disorder.

Hairy cell leukaemia behaves in an indolent manner and responds well to treatment with single-agent drugs such as 2-chlorodeoxyadenosine (cladribine) or pentostatin. Splenectomy and α-interferon are also effective treatment strategies.

The immunophenotype is CD20+ve, CD5-ve, sIg+ve, CD25+ve and CD11c+ve.

Diffuse large B-cell lymphoma

Diffuse large B-cell lymphoma (DLBC) is the commonest high-grade lymphoma. It typifies an aggressive but potentially curable lymphoma, and represents approximately one third of all lymphomas. Histologically, the disorder is characterized by the presence of sheets of large cells of B-cell origin. The disorder probably includes a variety of different can induce remission in approximately 80% of cases, and as many as 60% of patients will attain a sustained remission beyond three years. The combination of cyclophosphamide, doxorubicin (*h*ydroxydaunorubicin), vincristine (*O*ncovin) and *p*rednisolone (CHOP) has been the gold standard against which other treatments are judged. The treatment is administered every three weeks for a total of six or eight courses on an outpatient basis. The addition of the anti-CD20 antibody rituximab to CHOP chemotherapy has improved survival rates so that the combination of rituximab and CHOP (R-CHOP) has become the standard of care for patients with DLBC lymphoma. This finding is particularly significant for those patients with low-risk disease (Figure 9.8).

Relapsed patients can be offered high-dose chemotherapy and peripheral blood stem-cell rescue (Chapter 12). Patients who have chemosensitive disease may benefit from this approach. Radiotherapy is often given to sites of bulky disease or residual masses after the completion of chemotherapy.

The immunophenotype is CD20+ve, CD79+ve, CD5-ve, CD23-ve, CD10-ve and sIgM+ve. The immunophenotype may also reflect the cell of origin, e.g. GC or ABC type.

Burkitt Lymphoma (BL)

Burkitt lymphoma presents as three main forms: endemic, sporadic and a type associated with immunodeficiency states. The endemic form mainly affects children in east Africa, presents with a jaw or a facial bone tumour and is nearly always positive for the Epstein–Barr virus (EBV). Infection with malaria is thought to play an important part in the pathogenesis of this form of BL, probably by chronic antigen stimulation. Sporadic BL occurs in the West, is only sometimes EBV positive and tends to present with extranodal disease, most commonly an abdominal mass but breast, gonadal, CNS and bone marrow are other commonly affected sites. BL also occurs in HIV-positive patients.

The unifying feature of all three of these types of Burkitt lymphoma is activation of the *MYC* oncogene, as described in Chapter 8. All cases have a translocation of the *MYC* gene on chromosome 8 to one of the immunoglobulin genes on chromosome 14, 22 or 2 – t(8;14), t(2;8) and t(8;22). The translocation brings the *MYC* gene under the control of the immunoglobulin enhancer.

The pathology is characteristic, with diffuse infiltration by small to medium B lymphoma cells, a very high proliferation rate ~100% and a high rate of apoptosis, which leads to the characteristic 'starry sky' appearance.

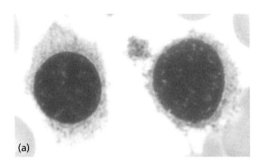

(a)

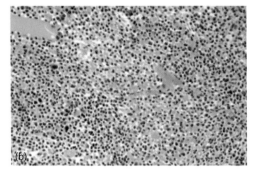

(b)

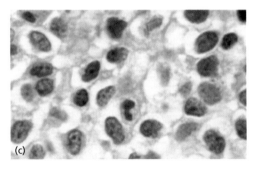

(c)

Figure 9.7 (a) Photomicrograph showing hairy cells in peripheral blood; (b) low-power view of trephine biopsy showing infiltration and hemorrhage; and (c) high-power view of trephine biopsy. The hairy cells have bean-shaped nuclei and abundant empty-looking cytoplasm (appearing like a halo around the nucleus).

lymphoma types and in this sense is a 'dustbin' for those lymphomas that do not obviously fit into other categories. At least two different types (ABC and GC types, see Chapter 8) of DLBCL have been identified based on gene expression profiling.

The disorder occurs at all ages, but becomes commoner in later life. Patients may present with night sweats, fever, weight loss and lymphadenopathy or with extranodal lymphoma involving sites such as the gastrointestinal tract, the testis, brain or bone. Treatment is with combination chemotherapy, which

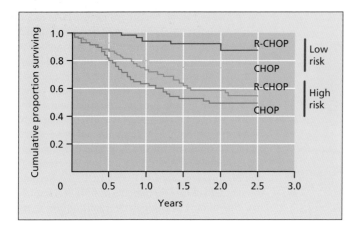

Figure 9.8 The survival of patients with DLBC lymphoma following treatment with CHOP alone, compared with CHOP plus rituximab (R-CHOP). Note that the survival difference is more pronounced for patients with low-risk disease.

The treatment of Burkitt lymphoma is generally a success story. Treatment with standard chemotherapy regimens such as CHOP leads to a poor prognosis, but since the introduction of multiagent sequential chemotherapy the outcome has been considerably improved. Patients with limited-stage disease have a >90% cure rate, while patients with more advanced disease can also be cured using this approach. CNS prophylactic treatment is necessary in all cases. The addition of rituximab has also been found to improve outcome.

The immunophenotype of Burkitt Lymphoma is of germinal centre type, CD19+ve, CD20+ve, BCL2-ve and CD10+ve.

Mucosa-associated lymphoid tissue lymphomas

The so-called mucosa-associated lymphoid tissue (MALT) lymphomas are typically extranodal, as their name suggests. This type of lymphoma belongs to the group of marginal zone lymphomas, as the malignant cells are thought to derive from the marginal zone of the lymphoid follicle. The commonest type is gastric MALT lymphoma. Patients usually present with a long history of indigestion and are found to have MALT lymphoma on gastric biopsy. Some, but by no means all, are associated with the presence of *Helicobacter pylori*. Eradication of the bacterium using combination antibiotic therapy often leads to eradication of the lymphoma. In those cases that cannot be treated successfully with antibiotics, gentle oral chemotherapy or involved field radiotherapy will usually control the disease. High-grade transformation may occur and is treated in the usual way with combination chemotherapy. Other common sites to be involved with this lymphoma include the thyroid gland, salivary glands, the lungs and the spleen.

The immunophenotype is CD20+ve, CD79+ve, CD5-ve, CD23-ve, CD10-ve and sIgM+ve.

AIDS-related lymphoma

Lymphoma is an AIDS-defining illness. Patients infected with HIV have a substantially increased risk of having lymphoma compared to the general population. The use of antiretroviral therapy has led to a decline in the incidence of AIDS-related non-Hodgkin lymphoma.

AIDS lymphoma is nearly always a B-cell neoplasm, most commonly of Burkitt's or diffuse large B-cell type. There is a propensity for involvement of extranodal sites, such as the gastrointestinal tract or the brain. Primary CNS lymphoma is a very rare finding in non-HIV-infected persons and HIV infection should be suspected in all such cases. AIDS-related lymphoma is a very aggressive disorder and the prognosis is generally poor. The use of antiretroviral therapy and combination chemotherapy has been reported to improve the prognosis.

Mycosis fungoides and Sezary syndrome

These disorders are T-cell cutaneous lymphomas. Mycosis fungoides is an indolent disorder characterized by plaques or nodules affecting the skin. The disorder can be controlled with PUVA and often waxes and wanes over many years. The disorder may eventually become systemic, and when this happens the prognosis is very poor. Sezary syndrome is characterized by generalized erythroderma and circulating abnormal lymphoid cells with cerebriform nuclei (Sezary cells) in the peripheral blood.

10

Myeloma and other paraproteinaemias

Learning objectives

✓ To understand the meaning of the term 'paraprotein' and to know the various clinical situations in which a paraprotein may be found

✓ To have a moderately detailed knowledge of the pathology, clinical features and diagnosis of myeloma and to understand the principles of treatment of this disorder

Multiple myeloma

Multiple myeloma is a disease arising from the malignant transformation of a terminally differentiated B cell (plasma cell). The differentiating cells of the malignant clone have the morphology of plasma cells or plasmacytoid lymphocytes, have clonally rearranged immunoglobulin genes (see pp. 60–62) and usually secrete a monoclonal immunoglobulin, IgG or IgA, a monoclonal light chain or both. Such monoclonal proteins are called paraproteins; they consist of structurally identical molecules and therefore produce a discrete monoclonal band (M band) on electrophoresis. The primary site of proliferation of the malignant plasma cells is the bone marrow (Figure 10.1). Activation of osteoclasts by molecules secreted from stromal cells, and the myeloma cells themselves, causes bone destruction that leads to multiple well-defined osteolytic lesions, radiological changes resembling those of generalized osteoporosis and hypercalcaemia. Marrow infiltration also causes impairment of haemopoiesis. Some patients with IgA paraproteins (which tend to dimerize) and a few patients with high levels of IgG3 paraproteins have a substantially raised plasma viscosity and may suffer from hyperviscosity syndrome. Light chains are filtered through the glomeruli and are found in the urine; they may damage the renal tubules. In 10% of patients, the abnormally folded paraprotein is converted into deposits of amyloid in various tissues. Levels of normal immunoglobulin are reduced and in advanced disease there is a reduction in circulating T cells. Extramedullary tumour deposits develop frequently.

Clinical features

The age-standardized incidence of myeloma is about 40 per million of the population per year. With an ageing population, approximately 4500 new cases are diagnosed each year. Most patients are between the ages of 50 and 80 years. In all cases there is a prolonged asymptomatic phase that may last for a number of years – so-called monoclonal gammopathy of undetermined significance (MGUS). As the

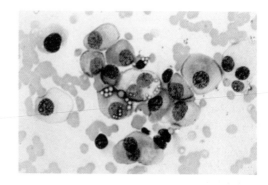

Figure 10.1 A marrow smear from a patient with multiple myeloma (May–Grünwald–Giemsa (MGG) stain).

Haematology Lecture Notes, Ninth edition. C.S.R. Hatton, N.C. Hughes-Jones, D. Hay and D. Keeling. © 2013 John Wiley & Sons, Ltd.
Published 2013 by John Wiley & Sons, Ltd.

disease advances and the bone marrow becomes infiltrated with malignant plasma cells secreting monoclonal immunoglobulin, a number of secondary changes may be found.

Bone destruction

The most common presenting symptom is bone pain, usually over the lumbar spine. Pathological fractures are frequent and often affect the lower thoracic and upper lumbar vertebrae and the ribs (Figure 10.2). Compression fractures of the vertebrae may damage the spinal cord or spinal roots and cause neurological symptoms. Large tumours may form in relation to any bone and cause pressure symptoms.

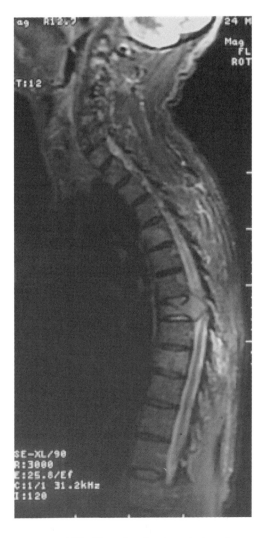

Figure 10.2 MRI of the spine showing spinal-cord compression secondary to myeloma.

Renal failure

Renal failure may be found at presentation or develop during the course of the disease. Chronic renal failure commonly results from the obstruction of distal renal tubules by proteinaceous casts, leading to tubular atrophy and interstitial fibrosis (myeloma kidney). Renal dysfunction may also result from the toxic effects of light chains on tubule cells, the deposition of light chains in glomeruli and amyloidosis. Acute renal failure may be precipitated by dehydration or use of analgesics, or be caused by hypercalcaemia or hyperuricaemia.

Bone marrow failure

Anaemia, neutropenia and thrombocytopenia may occur. The anaemia is usually normocytic or macrocytic. Mucosal bleeding is a common symptom and is due to interference with fibrin polymerization and platelet function. Platelet counts may be low in advanced cases.

Bacterial infections

Respiratory tract infections are common in patients with myeloma. The lack of normal antibodies (acquired hypogammaglobulinaemia) results in infections caused by capsulated organisms, commonly *pneumococcus* and *haemophilus*. Thus, pneumonia and sinusitis are common presentations.

Hypercalcaemia

Hypercalcaemia causes symptoms such as anorexia, vomiting, lethargy, stupor or coma. Patients may present more acutely with polyuria and polydipsia.

Amyloidosis

Peripheral neuropathy, macroglossia, cardiomegaly, diarrhoea and carpal tunnel syndrome suggest amyloidosis. Peripheral neuropathy may also be caused by infiltration of nerves by plasma cells or by a direct toxic effect of the paraprotein.

Hyperviscosity syndrome

This is characterized by neurological disturbances (dizziness, somnolence and coma), cardiac failure and haemorrhagic manifestations (Figure 10.3). IgA myeloma is more likely to cause hyperviscosity, as IgA has a tendency to form dimers.

Laboratory findings

A normochromic, normocytic or macrocytic anaemia is common. When the disease is advanced,

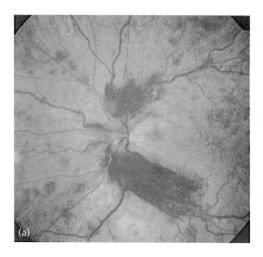

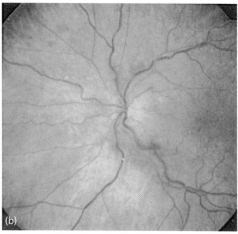

Figure 10.3 Fundi of the eyes in the hyperviscosity syndrome showing retinal haemorrhages (a) and papilloedema (b).

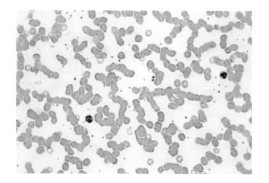

Figure 10.4 Blood film from a patient with multiple myeloma showing marked red cell rouleau formation (MGG stain).

thrombocytopenia and neutropenia may also be found. The blood film may show a leucoerythroblastic picture (reflecting marrow infiltration) and, in occasional patients, plasma cells; red cells may show an increased tendency to form rouleaux (Figure 10.4) and the paraprotein may cause an increased basophilic staining of the background between the red cells. The erythrocyte sedimentation rate (ESR) is often raised, frequently to more than 100 mm/hr. The serum uric acid is raised in about half of cases (and may contribute to the renal damage).

Bone marrow aspirates usually contain a greatly increased proportion of plasma cells (Figures 10.1 and 10.5(a). Some aspirates may show only a slight increase in plasma cells (5–10% of nucleated marrow

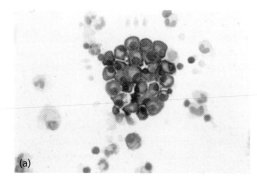

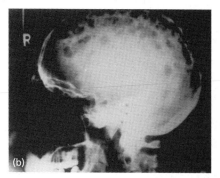

Figure 10.5 (a) Marrow smear showing myeloma cells reacting with antibody against λ-chains; the reaction was demonstrated using an immunoalkaline phosphatase method. The cells did not react with antibody against κ-chains and were therefore monoclonal in origin. The serum contained an IgD λ paraprotein. (b) Radiograph of the skull of a patient with multiple myeloma showing multiple discrete osteolytic lesions with no sclerosis at the margin.

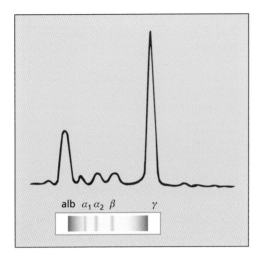

Figure 10.6 Illustration of serum electrophoresis demonstrating a monoclonal band and reduced normal immunoglobulins. *Source*: Courtesy of Professor Hoffbrand.

cells, as compared with 0.1–2% in normal marrow) and others may show no increase. The latter results from the multifocal nature of the plasma cell infiltrate.

Electrophoresis of serum usually demonstrates the monoclonal Ig as a discrete band (M band; Figure 10.6) and the nature of the paraprotein can be determined by immunofixation. Light chains (also called Bence-Jones proteins) can be detected in the serum and the urine using the sensitive 'free lite assay'. In 50% of patients with myeloma, the paraprotein is IgG, in 25% it is IgA, in 20% it is light chain only, and in 1–2% it is IgD or IgE. IgM-producing myelomas are extremely rare. Over half of patients with an IgG- or IgA-secreting myeloma have monoclonal light chains in their urine; in two-thirds of these patients the light chain is κ and in the remainder it is λ. In 1–2% of patients with myeloma, a paraprotein cannot be detected in either serum or concentrated urine (non-secretory myeloma).

Serum levels of β_2-microglobulin (the light chain of the HLA class 1 glycoproteins) correlates with tumour mass and, together with the serum albumin, is a very important prognostic marker (see below).

Diagnosis

This is often based on the finding of at least two of the following three features:

1 A monoclonal Ig in the serum or monoclonal light chains in the urine or both.
2 An increased proportion of plasma cells (often with atypical features) in marrow aspirates.

3 Discrete osteolytic lesions on X-ray studies (Figure 10.5(b)).

The differential diagnosis is from a benign paraproteinaemia (p. 91).

Treatment

Treatment should be reserved for patients in whom there is evidence of organ damage, for instance bone marrow infiltration, lytic or other bone lesions or renal dysfunction. Some patients may fulfil the diagnostic criteria of myeloma but have indolent or smouldering disease with stable paraproteins, and in the absence of lytic bone lesions or other end-organ damage no treatment is required. Treatment requires a multidisciplinary approach involving haematologists/oncologists and an extensive multidisciplinary team.

Supportive care measures are very important. Anaemia is a common finding at presentation or at progression or may be secondary to treatment, and patients who require frequent transfusion may benefit from subcutaneous erythropoietin. Adequate hydration and a good urine flow must be maintained in an attempt to reduce the risk of paraprotein precipitation in the renal tubules and consequent renal damage; haemodialysis may be required in the event of renal failure. Patients with high paraprotein levels may also develop hyperviscosity syndrome and plasma exchange can be used to reduce rapidly the effect of this problem. Bacterial infections, due to the associated acquired hypogammaglobulinaemia, require prompt treatment with antibiotics. Bone pain and fractures and hypercalcaemia cause significant morbidity and mortality in patients with myeloma. Long-term therapy with bisphosphonates has been shown to reduce bone pain and progression of skeletal lesions.

Chemotherapy

Cytotoxic drugs are reserved for patients with bone lesions, hypercalcaemia, bone marrow failure or renal dysfunction. Patients unable to receive high-dose therapy because of co-morbidities are usually treated with the alkylating drugs melphalan or cyclophosphamide, which can be given orally with or without prednisolone, either intermittently (for 4–5 days every 4 weeks) or in smaller doses, continuously. Recently, the addition of thalidomide has been shown to increase the response rate and the combination of melphalan, prednisolone and thalidomide (MPT) has become the standard of care for less fit, usually older patients who are not eligible for high-dose therapy and stem-cell rescue. The mechanism of action of thalidomide is unknown, but there is evidence to suggest that it may have antiangiogenic effects in myeloma. However, it has a number of troublesome side effects, including drowsiness, constipation, risk of thrombosis and peripheral neuropathy, in addition to its well-known teratogenicity.

Approximately 75–80% of patients respond to MPT, with an improvement in symptoms, a rise in haemoglobin and a reduction in the paraprotein level. The response is gradual and may take many months. Treatment reduces the tumour mass and is usually stopped when the paraprotein level ceases to fall (plateau phase).

In patients with a good performance status and minimal co-morbidities, chemotherapy programmes are undergoing a period of revision. The goals of treatment are changing from merely reducing the tumour burden to achieving a complete response and long-term remission, as determined by the disappearance of paraprotein levels and a complete reversal of end-organ damage. Newer drugs such as proteosome inhibitors (e.g. bortezomib) and thalidomide analogues such as lenalidomide are being added to conventional chemotherapy agents to reduce the tumour burden before consolidating with high-dose melphalan and stem cell rescue (Chapter 13). Response rates have been found to be very high and some patients are achieving durable remissions. This treatment is not curative, with over 90% of patients relapsing, but for patients able to tolerate this intensity of therapy there is evidence that it improves overall survival.

Radiotherapy

Radiotherapy is a very effective treatment for bone pain in myeloma. Spinal cord compression due to a vertebral or a paravertebral mass requires urgent assessment, and decompression laminectomy followed by radiotherapy is usually the treatment of choice. Bone fractures, which are a common complication, are best treated by orthopaedic fixation followed by radiotherapy.

Relapsed and refractory disease

Nearly all patients with myeloma will relapse after the initial therapy. Occasional patients have been cured with allogeneic bone marrow transplantation, but the technique is only suitable for patients under 45 years and carries a high mortality (Chapter 12). New agents continue to be developed for the treatment of relapsed myeloma. Bortezomib is a novel drug that inhibits the activity of the proteasome, the organelle responsible for regulated intracellular proteolysis. This agent has shown responses in 30–40% of patients with relapsed myeloma, probably by preventing the

degradation of IkB by the proteasome. IkB neutralizes NFkB, a molecule that drives cell proliferation.

Other treatment options available for relapsed myeloma include the use of the thalidomide analogue lenalidomide, or the oral alkylating agent melphalan. Second-generation proteasome inhibitor carfilzomib and pomalidomide, another thalidomide analogue, show promise in clinical trials and may be available for relapsed patients in the future. Palliative care services need to be involved for expert advice on pain control and management of specific symptoms.

Prognosis

The median survival from diagnosis is 4–5 years. Patients presenting with renal failure have a worse prognosis. Patients can be stratified according to the levels of serum β_2-microglobulin (a reflection of tumour burden and renal function) and albumin levels. High levels of β_2-microglobulin and low levels of albumin confer a poor prognosis. Certain cytogenetic abnormalities also provide prognostic information. Patients with high-risk cytogenetic features including deletion 17p and translocations t(14;16) or t(4;14) have a worse outcome.

Solitary plasmacytoma

Solitary tumours consisting of malignant plasma cells may be found in the bone marrow or in extramedullary sites such as the upper respiratory tract. It is common to find a monoclonal Ig in the serum or monoclonal light chains in the urine, or both. In the case of extramedullary plasmacytomas, there is often no evidence of tumour elsewhere and the prognosis after excision followed by local radiotherapy is very good.

Other paraproteinaemias and related disorders

Benign paraproteinaemia (benign monoclonal gammopathy or monoclonal gammopathy of undetermined significance, MGUS)

A paraprotein is found in the serum in 0.1–1.0% of normal adults and in up to 10% of elderly subjects. A high proportion of such individuals have a condition termed 'benign paraproteinaemia' that does not require treatment. The most important difference between MGUS and myeloma is the absence of end-organ damage in the former. However, MGUS will transform

Table 10.1 **The differences between myeloma and MGUS.**

	Myeloma	MGUS
Bone marrow plasma cells	>10% on bone marrow aspirate	<10% on bone marrow aspirate
Serum paraprotein	Usually high and rising	Usually low and stable
Bence–Jones proteinuria	>50% of cases	Rare
Immune paresis	Very common	Rare
Lytic bone lesions	Common	Absent
Hypercalcaemia	Common	Absent
Anaemia	Frequent	Absent
Impaired renal function	May be present	Absent

Note: Treatment is not indicated for patients with MGUS. Randomized trials have thus far demonstrated no benefit from early intervention and simple monitoring of the paraprotein with clinical review is all that is required.

to myeloma at the rate of 1% per year, emphasizing the importance of monitoring patients with an apparently benign paraproteinaemia. The differences between myeloma and MGUS are illustrated in Table 10.1.

Amyloidosis

Amyloidosis is a disorder of protein folding whereby normally soluble proteins are deposited as β-pleated sheets. Infiltration of organs with amyloid leads to dysfunction and eventual organ failure. Amyloid may be demonstrated in rectal, gingival or renal biopsies; it stains positively with Congo red and shows an apple green birefringence in polarized light. Amyloid may be one of three principal types:

1 *AA amyloid*: Seen in patients with long-term chronic infections or inflammatory disorders. The amyloid protein is derived from serum amyloid A-related protein. This protein is synthesized in inflammatory states and, if present for long enough at a high enough level, becomes deposited in various organs.
2 *AL amyloid*: These proteins consist of part or whole of the immunoglobulin light chain. The classical features include macroglossia, carpal tunnel syndrome, peripheral neuropathy and purpura, but more important clinically are malabsorption, nephrotic syndrome and cardiomyopathy. Patients are found to have monoclonal light chain excretion. They may have an increased number of plasma cells in the bone marrow but do not have bone lesions. Few effective treatment modalities exist and prognosis is therefore poor (especially in patients with cardiac infiltration). Where treatment is given it is usually derived from the protocols used for patients with myeloma.

3 *Familial forms*: This is a diverse group of diseases, often presenting as neuropathy but frequently involving other organs.

Waldenström's macroglobulinaemia (see Chapter 9, p. 82)

Waldenström's macroglobulinaemia (or lymphoplasmacytic lymphoma) is also characterized by the presence of a paraprotein, although, in contrast to myeloma, in this condition it is nearly always IgM. The IgM paraprotein is secreted by a clonal population of pleomorphic lymphocytes and plasma cells that infiltrate the bone marrow, lymph nodes and spleen. Symptoms result both from tissue infiltration and from hyperviscosity of the blood caused by high levels of IgM. Osteolytic lesions are rare. It is a relatively uncommon condition, being found at approximately 10% of the incidence of myeloma.

Heavy chain diseases

In these rare paraproteinaemias, the B lineage-derived malignant clone secretes γ, α or μ heavy chains rather than complete Ig molecules. The clinical picture is that of a lymphoma; α-chain disease is characterized by severe malabsorption due to infiltration of the small intestine by lymphoma cells.

Other lymphoproliferative disorders

A paraprotein may also be found in chronic cold haemagglutinin disease, and in some patients with malignant lymphoma or chronic lymphocytic leukaemia.

11

Neoplastic disorders of myeloid cells

Learning objectives

✓ To understand the presentation, natural history and diagnosis of acute myeloblastic leukaemia

✓ To have an understanding of the myelodysplastic disorders

✓ To be familiar with the term myeloproliferative disorder and the four main types – chronic myeloid leukaemia, polycythaemia vera, myelofibrosis and essential thrombocythaemia

✓ To appreciate the expanding scientific understanding of these conditions

---

Myeloid cells include granulocytic-neutrophil, eosinophil, monocyte and basophil precursors, erythroid and megakaryocytic cell lineages, all of which are thought to arise from a single multipotent common stem cell. The earliest morphologically recognizable cell in the granulocytic lineage is called the myeloblast. The myeloblast differentiates to become a promyelocyte with the appearance of azurophilic granules. Further maturation sees the appearance of specific granules and the disappearance of blast-like features. The cells at this stage are known as myelocytes, eosinophil myelocytes, basophil myelocytes and neutrophil myelocytes. The neutrophil myelocyte divides and the progeny develop into metamyelocytes and finally mature neutrophils, as outlined on pp. 3, 4. These later stages are characterized by the involution of the nucleus as it becomes less spherical and more band-like. Monocytes are derived from promonocytes that are recognizable morphologically. The earliest erythroid cell that can be identified morphologically within the bone marrow is the proerythroblast. These large cells with dark blue cytoplasm mature and divide to become normoblasts, reticulocytes and finally mature red cells. Megakaryocytes are large, multinucleated cells that derive from megakaryoblasts, which give rise to platelets by cytoplasmic shedding (Chapter 1).

A neoplastic clone can emerge from any of these stages, although the more mature cells are less often involved in the neoplastic process. The malignant process may be obvious, with large numbers of blast cells – *acute myeloid leukaemia (AML)*. Other disorders can be divided, with some overlap, into *myelodysplastic* and *myeloproliferative* conditions. The myelodysplastic disorders are characterized by abnormal morphology (dysplasia) with altered function; there is often an excess of blast cells, the abnormalities terminating as a florid leukaemia. The myeloproliferative disorders are characterized by increased numbers of cells with relatively normal morphology and function. The myeloproliferative disorders may also transform to acute leukaemia, but this is an uncommon event.

Acute myeloid leukaemia

AML is a clonal disorder of myeloid progenitor cells that may occur at any age, but becomes increasingly common in older people. It is the most common form of acute leukaemia in adults. The disorder leads to an infiltration of the bone marrow, with immature cells resulting in impaired production of neutrophils,

---

Haematology Lecture Notes, Ninth edition. C.S.R. Hatton, N.C. Hughes-Jones, D. Hay and D. Keeling. © 2013 John Wiley & Sons, Ltd. Published 2013 by John Wiley & Sons, Ltd.

platelets and red cells. Blast cells frequently appear in the peripheral blood and may derive from any of the lineages described above. The classification of the disorder is based on morphology, cytogenetics, immunophenotyping and clinical behaviour, reminiscent of the classification of lymphoid disorders.

Aetiology

The vast majority of cases have no identifiable aetiology, although a number of cases may evolve from other clonal myeloid disorders such as the myelodysplastic disorders and the myeloproliferative conditions. Radiation and benzene exposure are also known to lead to AML. There are rare incidences when individuals have a predisposition to AML. Children affected with Down's syndrome have a 400 times higher incidence of acute megakaryocytic leukaemia (M7) compared with unaffected children. In addition, there are families that have inherited mutations of critical haematopoietic transcription factors (e.g. AML-1) that may give rise to AML.

Classification

The malignant cells are thought to represent neoplastic equivalents of normal maturation stages and eight types are covered by the well-recognized FAB classification:

1 Undifferentiated blasts: M0
2 Lightly granulated blasts: M1
3 Granulated blasts often with Auer rods: M2
4 Promyelocytic leukaemia: M3
5 Myelomonocytic leukaemia: M4
6 Monocytic leukaemia: M5
7 Erythroleukaemia: M6
8 Megakaryocytic leukaemia: M7

Previous attempts at classifying AML have been based on the morphological features described above. However, as the underlying molecular abnormalities that give rise to AML become better understood, attempts are being made to produce a more scientifically coherent classification. The WHO classification therefore attempts to classify AML by its underlying molecular abnormalities (e.g. recurrent cytogenetic changes). The complexities of this new classification, given in Table 11.1, reflect our incomplete knowledge of the molecular basis in many cases of AML.

Symptoms and signs

The clinical features reflect the consequences of *bone marrow failure*. Thus, anaemia causes pallor,

Table 11.1 **WHO 2001 classification of AML.**

Acute myeloblastic leukaemia with recurrent cytogenetic changes	AML with t(8;21); inv16 t(15;17); all mostly occurring in young patients
AML with multilineage dysplasia	Evolving from a myelodysplastic disorder; mostly occurring in older patients
AML and MDS, therapy related	Alkylating agent related, topoisomerase II inhibitor related
AML not otherwise categorized	Morphologically classified M0–M7 as previously according to cell of origin

Notes: AML – acute myeloid leukaemia; MDS – myelodysplastic syndromes.

tiredness and exertional dyspnoea; leucopenia leads to infection; and thrombocytopenia causes bleeding, bruising and purpura. Blast cells may infiltrate other organs such as the skin or gums (particularly in monocytic leukaemia), and there may be lymph adenopathy and splenomegaly. Massive splenomegaly is unusual in this disorder. Blast cells can invade the CNS, although this is commoner at relapse.

Laboratory findings

Laboratory findings, like the clinical findings, reflect bone marrow failure. Anaemia results from inadequate red cell production. Thrombocytopenia is nearly always present and results both from a failure of production and from increased consumption. Some cases of AML are associated with disseminated intravascular coagulation (DIC). The white cell count may be very high, reflecting the high circulating blast-cell count, but in about half of patients the total white cell count is low. In almost all cases the total number of normal circulating neutrophils is reduced.

The bone marrow always contains blast cells, sometimes accounting for more than 90% of the nucleated cells (Figure 11.1).

AML must be distinguished from acute lymphoblastic leukaemia (ALL), because their treatment and management differ. The morphological features may be diagnostic, but in cases where the blast cells are not well differentiated and lack granules, the cytochemical demonstration of certain intracellular enzymes or expression of a typical antigen profile by immunophenotyping may be required. *Auer rods* are needle-shaped or rod-shaped cytoplasmic inclusions

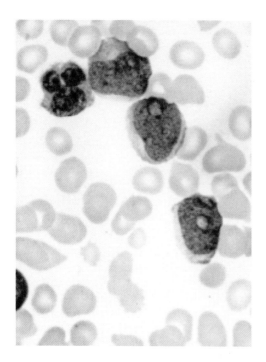

Figure 11.1 AML (FAB category M1). The three leukaemic myeloblasts are considerably larger than adjacent red cells, have finely stippled nuclear chromatin and show prominent nucleoli (MGG (May–Grünwald–Giemsa) stain).

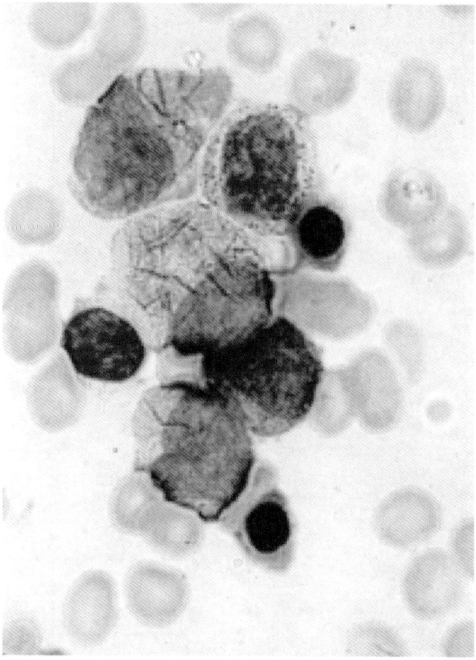

Figure 11.2 Myeloblasts of AML showing several Auer rods (MGG stain). These are azurophilic rod-shaped cytoplasmic inclusions that are exclusively found in some of the leukaemic myeloblasts of a small proportion of patients with AML, or CML in blast-cell transformation.

(formed by fusion of granules) within blast cells and are virtually diagnostic of AML (Figure 11.2).

Immunophenotyping using flow cytometry is a method whereby the antigen profile of the leukaemic cells can be identified (see Chapter 5 and Figure 11.3). Myeloid antigens such as CD13, CD15, CD33, the stem cell marker CD34 and stem cell factor receptor c-kit (CD117) help to identify blast cells as myeloid rather than lymphoid. The lymphoblasts in ALL will express B- or T-cell markers. In rare cases, leukaemias express both myeloid and lymphoid antigens and these are classified as biphenotypic leukaemias.

AML with recurrent genetic abnormalities

A number of characteristic cytogenetic abnormalities occur in AML. Their importance in terms of causation is becoming increasingly clear, and it is also now well established that certain abnormalities are associated with useful prognostic information (Table 11.2). For example, AML with t(8;21) or inv16 is associated with a more favourable prognosis.

In addition to these 'classic' cytogenetic abnormalities, research is uncovering additional mutations of prognostic significance. Mutations of a cytokine receptor (FLT-3) are thought to impart an adverse prognosis in some subtypes of AML. In some series up to 30% of cases carry such mutations. Abnormal localization of mutated nucleophosmin (NPM1) is present in half of cytogenetically normal AML and is associated with a better prognosis. Current research has uncovered point mutations in critical haemopoietic transcription factors (CEBPA and core binding factor, CBF). The prevalence and clinical significance of these mutations are still a matter of research, but it is hoped that some mutations will be predictive of prognosis and will influence management.

Therapy-related AML has been recognized as a late complication of chemotherapy. In these patients there is a recurring abnormality of chromosome 5 and/or 7 (25/del(5q) or 27/del(7q)). Patients who have received topoisomerase II inhibitors (etoposide) have a high incidence of balanced translocations involving 11q23 and 21q22. Therapy-related AML has a very poor prognosis.

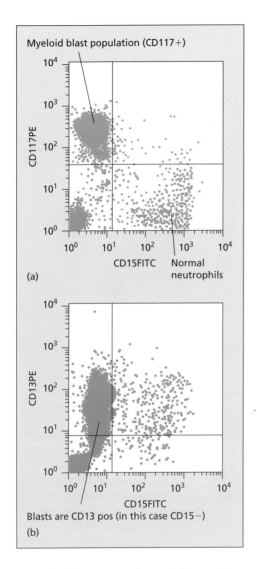

(a)

(b)

Figure 11.3 Flow cytometry demonstrating myeloid antigen expression in a case of AML. The blasts are CD117+ and CD13+.

Acute promyelocytic leukaemia (M3)

This variant deserves special mention, not only because it has specific clinical manifestations but also because of the molecular understanding of the disorder. The malignant cells in acute promyelocytic leukaemia (APML) are promyelocytes that contain abundant granules and numerous Auer rods. Release of the promyelocytes' granules, which may occur spontaneously or at the initiation of cytotoxic therapy, is known to produce uncontrolled activation of

Table 11.2 **Cytogenetic abnormalities that have been found to be associated with better prognosis in AML.**	
Translocation t(8;21)	Found in granulocytic variant of AML; the blast cells have obvious granules and Auer rods are frequently present
Translocation t(15;17)	Defines acute promyelocytic leukaemia (APML). The leukaemic promyelocytes are heavily granulated with prominent Auer rods. This type is associated with a severe coagulopathy
Inversion Inv(16)	Occurs in myelomonocytic leukaemia with an excess of eosinophils in the bone marrow

the fibrinolytic system. The result is DIC and potentially life-threatening bleeding.

Treatment with all-trans-retinoic acid (ATRA) allows differentiation of the abnormal promyelocytes and limits the threat of DIC. This differentiating agent alone allows some patients to reach remission, although most will subsequently relapse. The combination of ATRA with conventional chemotherapy has made APML the most curable subtype of AML.

The molecular basis of APML and the sensitivity of the disorder to ATRA are of considerable interest. The disorder is characterized by a translocation between chromosome 15 and chromosome 17. The breakpoint on chromosome 17 falls within the gene for the retinoic acid receptor ($RAR\alpha$), which is normally needed for appropriate differentiation of the cell. The breakpoint on chromosome 15 falls within the gene known as PML, a nuclear regulatory factor needed to control the induction of apoptosis of the cell. As a result of the translocation, a new fusion gene called PML-RAR-α is produced, which encodes a DNA-binding protein, causing a maturation block. This can be overcome by pharmacological doses of ATRA. Patients with APML can therefore be very effectively treated with ATRA (differentiating agent), together with chemotherapy. The prognosis for this rare subtype has improved dramatically with the use of this approach.

Treatment of AML

The treatment of AML can be divided into four main components: intensive chemotherapy, supportive care, differentiation agents and bone marrow transplantation (BMT).

Intensive chemotherapy

The use of anthracycline drugs together with cytosine arabinoside leads to remissions in up to 80%

of younger patients. Following administration of chemotherapy, there is a disappearance of circulating blast cells and a temporary worsening of the cytopenias, leading to severe neutropenia and thrombocytopenia. Elderly patients have lower rates of remission and generally have a poor prognosis: patients over 70 years of age rarely survive beyond one year due to resistant disease or to complications of therapy.

Supportive care

Following chemotherapy, there is an inevitable period of neutropenia associated with a breakdown of mucosal surfaces; patients commonly complain of a sore throat and dysphagia and may develop abdominal pain as a result of inflammation of the bowel mucosa. This is the period when the patient is susceptible to overwhelming septicaemia (neutropenic sepsis); the infection most often arises from damaged mucosal surfaces of the gut, in particular the large bowel, allowing the passage of Gram-negative organisms into the bloodstream. The presence of fever or other features of infection should lead to prompt administration of intravenous antibiotics aimed at Gram-negative organisms. The intensity of the chemotherapy used to treat AML may lead to periods of neutropenia continuing for as long as three to four weeks. Such extended periods of neutropenia are associated with fungal infection, notably invasive *Aspergillus* and *Candida* species. Prophylactic antifungal treatment helps reduce *Candida* infection. Platelet and red cell transfusions are necessary until normal haematopoiesis is restored. Additional courses of chemotherapy will reduce the blast count still further and can lead to durable remissions in a significant number of cases.

Bone marrow transplantation (see Chapter 12)

For patients with features indicating poor-risk disease or who have relapsed, BMT may be curative. Allogeneic BMT relies on using myeloablative therapy (which may involve treatment with either drugs alone or a combination of drugs and radiotherapy); it aims to destroy the patient's bone marrow and considerably reduce the number of malignant blast cells. Immunosuppression allows the HLA-matched donor bone marrow to engraft, usually in two to three weeks. The donor marrow can then induce a 'graft versus leukaemia effect', an immunological effect that eradicates chemoresistant disease. Historically, the use of myeloablative allogeneic BMT has been restricted to younger patients (aged <45 years) because of the severe toxicity associated with the procedure. More

recently, reduced intensity (non-myeloablative) protocols for allogeneic BMT have been developed allowing the graft versus leukaemia effect to be harnessed for older patients (45–70 years).

The myelodysplastic syndromes

The myelodysplastic syndromes (MDS) are serious, relatively common disorders in which the bone marrow is populated by a clone of abnormal haemopoietic cells. These cells are dysplastic and are unable to mature normally. The maturation block tends to worsen over time, leading to an accumulation of blast cells and ultimately the disorder may lead to bone marrow failure, either as a result of a transformation to acute leukaemia or because of stem cell failure. The marrow blast-cell count is the single most important factor in determining prognosis, with a higher blast count conferring a poorer prognosis. The disease is most common in the elderly and is rare before the age of 50 years. MDS presents most commonly with symptoms of anaemia, but infection, bruising or bleeding may also occur. MDS has been subdivided into a number of categories depending on the presence of underlying cytogenetic abnormalities and morphological features such as ring sideroblasts.

Laboratory features

Typically, there is reduction in at least two cell lines (e.g. anaemia and leucopenia, or anaemia and thrombocytopenia). The anaemia is frequently macrocytic (not due to vitamin B12 or folate deficiency) and the neutrophils are 'dysplastic' – they look bizarre, often with reduced granulation and abnormal nuclear maturation, including the characteristic bilobed spectacle-like nuclei (Figure 11.4). Blasts cells may be found in the peripheral blood. An increase in peripheral blood monocytes ($>1 \times 10^9$/L) in some cases defines these patients as having *chronic myelomonocytic leukaemia* (CMML).

The bone marrow has variable cellularity, although there is always abnormal maturation recognized by microscopy. The blast count may vary from less than 5% in *refractory anaemia* (RA) to more than 5% blasts in *refractory anaemia with excess blasts* (RAEB). A blast-cell count greater than 20% in the bone marrow defines the condition as acute leukaemia. The presence of iron granules in the mitochondria of erythroid precursors (nucleated red cells), forming a ring of iron-positive granules around the nucleus, defines the condition known as *primary acquired*

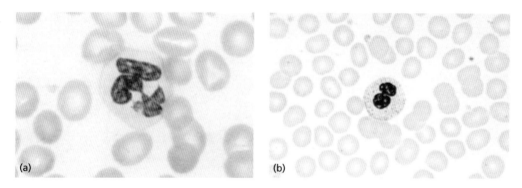

Figure 11.4 (a) Hypogranular neutrophil from a patient with MDS. (b) Neutrophil granulocyte from a heterozygote for the inherited Pelger–Huët anomaly. The nucleus is bilobed (spectacle-like) and has markedly condensed chromatin. In heterozygotes for this asymptomatic condition, 50–70% of neutrophils show these changes. Similar abnormalities may be found in some neutrophils, as an acquired condition in MDS.

sideroblastic anaemia or *refractory anaemia with ring sideroblasts* (RARS). Cytogenetic abnormalities occur in about 50% of MDS cases.

Treatment

Treatment is usually supportive only, as this condition responds poorly to chemotherapy. Many patients are transfusion dependent. In younger patients, chemotherapy and BMT may be the treatment of choice. Trials have shown that certain growth factors such as erythropoietin and granulocyte stimulatory agents (G-CSF) can alleviate the associated cytopenias in certain subgroups of patients with MDS. Other subgroups of MDS have been shown to respond to the immunomodulatory agent lenalidamide, although the mechanism is not understood. The DNA hypomethylating agent azacitidine has also been shown to confer a modest survival benefit in patients with RAEB.

Myeloproliferative disorders

The myeloproliferative disorders are a group of diseases in which there is increased proliferative activity with fairly normal maturation, unlike MDS. Functional abnormalities of the blood cells are usually mild, but there may be an increase in the numbers of neutrophils, erythrocytes or platelets.

The myeloproliferative disorders are chronic myeloid leukaemia (CML), polycythaemia vera, myelofibrosis and essential thrombocythaemia.

Chronic myeloid leukaemia

CML is very rare in children, but increases in incidence with age. The most frequent symptoms are fatigue, weight loss, sweats and anorexia. The commonest signs are pallor and sometimes massive splenomegaly. Very occasionally CML may present with symptoms of hyperviscosity due to a very high white cell count. Priapism, tinnitus and stupor are among the commoner symptoms of this presentation.

Laboratory features

The peripheral blood abnormalities are characteristic. Patients are almost always anaemic and have elevated white cell counts (usually between 50 and 400×10^9/L), with excess neutrophils, myelocytes, metamyelocytes and basophils present in the peripheral blood (Figure 11.5); blast cells are also present in small numbers (usually <10%). The bone marrow is very hypercellular, with greatly increased white cell production.

Clinical course

The disorder runs a predictable course. In the first phase (the '*chronic phase*'), normal blood counts are achieved with therapy and the patient is generally well. This phase may continue for many years. Inevitably the disease then transforms through an *accelerated phase* (blood counts become difficult to control) into *blast crisis*. This latter phase is defined by an increasing number of blasts in the bone marrow, and in terms of its natural history is akin to acute leukaemia. Symptomatically, patients describe weight loss, night sweats and fevers. Some patients in blast crisis may

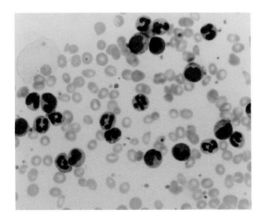

Figure 11.5 Blood film from a patient with CML showing an increased number of white cells, mainly neutrophils, band cells and metamyelocytes. Note the presence of some myelocytes and basophils.

be rescued with conventional chemotherapy and enter a second chronic phase.

Philadelphia chromosome

CML is associated with a pathognomonic chromosomal rearrangement in which there is a reciprocal translocation between chromosome 22 and chromosome 9. This leads to the formation of a novel gene that is transcribed into a novel oncoprotein with tyrosine kinase activity (BCR–ABL; Figure 11.6(a)). This protein leads to increased cell cycling and a failure of apoptosis. The fusion chromosome 22q– (with additional material from chromosome 9) is known as the *Philadelphia chromosome*. In 1990, two experimental approaches demonstrated the ability of the *BCR-ABL* fusion gene (as the sole abnormality) to cause leukaemia. First, transgenic mice that express the *BCR-ABL* gene have been shown to develop a rapidly fatal acute leukaemia; second, when murine bone marrow cells transfected with a *BCR-ABL* expressing retrovirus

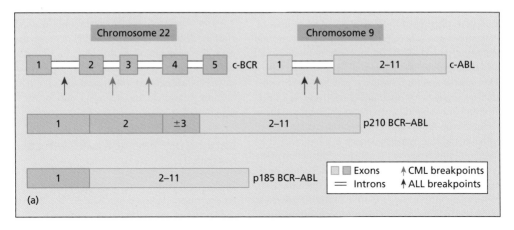

(a)

Figure 11.6 (a) Illustration of the translocation between chromosomes 22 and 9 leading to the formation of a novel oncogene *BCR–ABL*. Note that a variation of the same translocation occurs in some patients with ALL. The novel oncogene produces a tyrosine kinase, leading to cell proliferation. (b) Diagram showing the mechanism of action of imatinib. This drug inhibits the phosphorylation by BCR–ABL of tyrosine in protein (shown in green) and thereby interferes with its leukaemogenic effects.

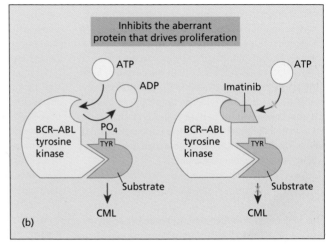

(b)

were used to repopulate the bone marrow of irradiated mice, the mice developed various myeloproliferative disorders, including CML.

These observations have led to the concept that the tyrosine kinase (TK) BCR–ABL is a target for therapy. Inhibitors of the ATP-binding site on this tyrosine kinase have therefore been developed to treat CML. The first such compound that emerged as a specific inhibitor of BCR–ABL was imatinib, a generally well tolerated oral agent that when taken daily can control the disease effectively for years (Figure 11.6(b)). Patients intolerant of imatinib can be treated with one of the newer tyrosine kinase inhibitors such as dasatinib or nilotinib. By blocking the inactive conformation of the BCR–ABL oncoprotein, TK inhibitors allow inhibition of its oncogenetic activity and thereby treat CML at the molecular level.

Treatment

The majority of patients with CML will respond to imatinib therapy with normalization of their blood counts and reduction of their enlarged spleens. Hydroxycarbamide is often used in the first few days to help reduce very high white cell counts, which are a common feature at presentation. The majority of patients will achieve a cytogenetic remission when treated with a TK inhibitor and many patients will remain in remission for many years. Imatinib is relatively well tolerated and only a handful of patients are resistant. Those patients who are resistant to imatinib can be treated with second-line tyrosine kinase inhibitors such as dasatinib, which targets the active conformation of the tyrosine kinase. TK inhibitors have successfully managed to delay the onset of blast transformation. CML provides an outstanding example of the effectiveness of targeted therapy, in which the understanding of molecular mechanisms has enabled the development of specific drugs to block offending oncogenic proteins.

While imatinib will provide control of CML in many cases, it cannot cure the disease. Allogeneic BMT is the only known curative therapy for this disorder and is most successfully carried out in the chronic phase. This procedure is not available to patients over the age of 45–50 years and relies on being able to identify a tissue-matched donor, either a sibling or an unrelated matched donor. The majority of patients with CML will not be found to have a suitable matched donor or will be too old for allogeneic BMT.

Polycythaemia vera

This chronic clonal disorder is characterized by excessive proliferation of a multipotent haemopoietic stem cell, resulting in an increased number of red cells, often accompanied by an increase in white cell and platelet counts. The primary clinical manifestation is markedly elevated haemoglobin and haematocrit. The clonal nature of the abnormal cells has been known for some time, but now a defining mutation in the erythropoietin signalling pathway (JAK2) has been identified. This mutation has been found in over 95% of cases of polycythaemia vera and JAK2 mutational analysis has become an important diagnostic test in this disorder.

Clinical features

Polycythaemia vera has an insidious onset, usually presenting late in life (rarely before 40 years). The main presenting symptoms relate to the considerable rise in red cell count and resulting increase in blood viscosity and include headache, dizziness and sometimes stroke. Pruritus, particularly after a hot bath, is a characteristic symptom. There is a marked tendency for patients to develop thrombosis, although there may also be an increased likelihood of bleeding. Mesenteric, portal or splenic vein thrombosis should alert the clinician to the possibility of polycythaemia vera. The principal signs are plethora (florid, dusky red colour of the face), splenomegaly and hepatomegaly. Erythromelalgia (increased skin temperature, burning sensation and redness) may occur in the extremities.

Laboratory findings and natural history

The red cell count and haemoglobin concentration are increased; haemoglobin values of 18–24 g/dL are common and the packed cell volume (PCV) is usually over 0.48 in females and 0.52 in males; the red cell mass (measured using ^{51}Cr-labelled red cells) is increased by over 25%. An increase in the white cell count occurs in many patients and about 50% of patients have an elevated platelet count.

Most patients with polycythaemia vera will remain well in the so-called plethoric phase, provided that the haematocrit is controlled to <45% by venesection. Furthermore, many patients can expect to have a normal life expectancy. Eventually the marrow may become increasingly fibrotic (myelofibrosis), leading to a fall in the haematocrit, increasing splenomegaly and often a requirement for blood transfusion in the later stages.

There are various cytogenetic abnormalities in the bone marrow cells of some cases, but no consistent abnormality has been detected.

Differential diagnosis

Secondary polycythaemia is the main differential diagnosis for polycythaemia vera. Longstanding hypoxia caused by cardiopulmonary disease or living at high altitudes will lead to an increased red cell mass and therefore a high haemoglobin and haematocrit (see Chapter 2). However, the elevated haematocrit and haemoglobin are usually the only haematological abnormality; where leucocytosis, thrombocytosis and splenomegaly are also found, polycythaemia vera is more likely. Some patients may have a high haematocrit as a result of a reduction in the plasma volume (e.g. due to diuretics). So-called *apparent polycythaemia* can be differentiated from polycythaemia vera and secondary polycythaemia by measurement of the red cell mass and the plasma volume. The JAK2 mutation, which characterizes nearly all cases of polycythaemia vera, is not present in secondary or apparent polycythaemia.

Treatment

The mainstay of treatment is venesection, aiming to lower the haematocrit below 0.50, and preferably below 0.45, thus preventing thrombotic episodes. In the early stages this may have to be performed at least twice weekly. Low-dose aspirin is also frequently used to minimize the risk of stroke. Patients with significant leucocytosis or thrombocytosis can be treated with cytoreductive therapy using oral chemotherapy agents such as hydroxycarbamide or busulphan. A single injection of radioactive phosphorus (^{32}P) can be very effective in controlling the red cell counts, but the significant risk of inducing secondary leukaemia has made this agent unpopular.

Primary myelofibrosis

This is a clonal disorder of the haematopoietic stem cell, which typically occurs after the age of 50 years. It is characterized by splenomegaly (which may be massive), immature circulating cells in the blood (nucleated red cells and myelocytes) and distorted red cells (so-called teardrop cells). These findings are due to the defining feature of myelofibrosis, bone marrow fibrosis. The marrow fibrosis is reactive and non-clonal and is thought to be secondary to the abnormal haemopoiesis, particularly of the megakaryocytic lineage. At the molecular level, approximately 50% of patients with primary myelofibrosis harbor the JAK2 mutation that has been identified in patients with primary polycythaemia. In other patients, mutations affecting the thrombopoietin receptor have been described. Many patients with an identical phenotype and with clonal haematopoiesis do not have either of these mutations and it is therefore impossible to know the full relevance of these findings to date.

The disorder may transform to acute leukaemia. Although the principal site of extramedullary haemopoiesis is the spleen or liver, other sites such as the lymph nodes, adrenal or dura may be involved.

Clinical features

This disorder usually presents in patients over the age of 50 years, but can occasionally occur in children. Patients may present with constitutional symptoms such as weight loss, night sweats or fever. Other presenting symptoms include splenic pain or symptoms due to anaemia such as fatigue, shortness of breath and palpitations. Occasional patients may present with gout as a consequence of hyperuricaemia resulting from the high cell turnover. Presenting signs include hepatomegaly, splenomegaly (nearly all cases) and pallor.

Laboratory findings

Normochromic normocytic anaemia is found in most patients with myelofibrosis. Leucocytosis and thrombocytosis are common findings, although the total white cell count is not usually as high as that found in CML and is rarely over 40×10^9/L. Inspection of the blood film is often diagnostic. The blood film typically shows the presence of normoblasts and myelocytes (i.e. a leucoerythroblastic picture, with the presence of teardrop poikilocytes; Figure 11.7). Bone marrow aspiration is often unsuccessful because of the

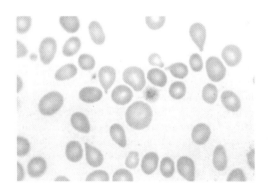

Figure 11.7 Blood film of a patient with idiopathic myelofibrosis showing several teardrop-shaped poikilocytes and an abnormally large platelet (MGG stain).

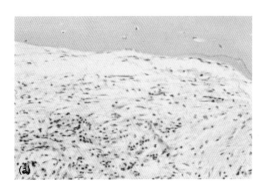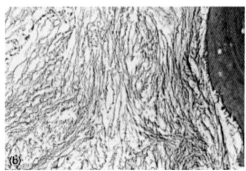

Figure 11.8 (a) Trephine biopsy of the bone marrow of a patient with idiopathic myelofibrosis showing fibroblasts and collagen fibrosis (haematoxylin and eosin). (b) Section of the same trephine biopsy showing increased reticulin fibres (silver impregnation of reticulin).

fibrosis, resulting in a dry tap. The bone marrow biopsy shows myeloproliferation with granulocytic and megakaryocytic hyperplasia together with fibrosis, which may be dense (Figure 11.8).

Treatment

Many patients need no specific treatment, but patients with a more proliferative marrow may require cytoreductive treatment with a gentle chemotherapy drug such as oral daily hydroxycarbamide. Monitoring of the patient's blood count is necessary in all cases. Most patients will become transfusion dependent and, as in the case of any patient requiring regular transfusion, iron loading of tissues may occur. Massive splenic enlargement can give rise to pain, which may necessitate splenectomy. Removal of the spleen may reduce transfusion requirements. The median survival of patients with myelofibrosis is in the order of five years from the time of diagnosis, but some patients may survive for many years. The only curative therapy for primary myelofibrosis is allogeneic stem-cell transplantation. A number of series have demonstrated the feasibility of reduced intensity conditioned allografting in high-risk patients. Clearly, many patients with this disorder will either be too old for stem-cell transplant or will have low-risk indolent disease. Causes of death in patients with primary myelofibrosis include infection, haemorrhage or transformation to acute leukaemia. More recently, JAK2 inhibitors such as ruxolitinib have been developed, which are effective at reducing the spleen size and improving constitutional symptoms in patients with myelofibrosis. While these molecularly targeted agents are effective at improving symptoms, similarly to imatinib in CML they are not curative.

Essential thrombocythaemia

This is a clonal myeloproliferative disorder that chiefly involves the megakaryocyte cell line. The disorder is classically associated with a marked rise in the platelet count, the haemoglobin concentration and the white cell count usually being unaffected. Many patients are diagnosed by the incidental finding of thrombocytosis during the course of a routine blood count. The difficulty arises in differentiating this condition from reactive causes of thrombocytosis (Table 11.3), as there is no specific diagnostic test for essential thrombocythaemia (Table 11.4). Approximately 50% of patients with ET have the common JAK2 mutation that has been identified in patients with primary polycythaemia and primary myelofibrosis. It is not yet clear how this single mutation can give rise to these three distinct disease entities.

Table 11.3 Causes of thrombocytosis.

Reactive

- Haemorrhage, haemolysis, trauma, surgery, postpartum, recovery from thrombocytopenia
- Acute and chronic infections
- Chronic inflammatory disease (e.g. ulcerative colitis, rheumatoid arthritis)
- Malignant disease (e.g. carcinoma, Hodgkin lymphoma, MDS)
- Splenectomy and splenic atrophy
- Iron-deficiency anaemia

Chronic myeloproliferative disorders

- Essential thrombocythaemia, polycythaemia vera, chronic myeloid leukaemia, idiopathic myelofibrosis

Table 11.4 Diagnostic criteria for essential thrombocythaemia.

- Platelet count over 500 × 10⁹/L (sustained)

- ET bone marrow changes – proliferation of megakaryocytes

- Does not meet criteria for diagnosis of polycythaemia vera, myelofibrosis, CML or MDS

- Presence of JAK2 mutation or other clonal marker

- In the absence of a clonal marker, no known cause for reactive thrombocytosis

Clinical features

This is a disorder that affects older patients, usually presenting with thrombotic or bleeding complications. Many patients are asymptomatic at presentation. Older patients seem to be at greater risk of thrombosis, particularly arterial. The main thrombotic complications are:

- Erythromelalgia and digital ischaemia. Erythromelalgia is characterized by intense burning and pain in the extremities. The pain is increased by exercise, warmth or dependency. The extremities are warm with mottled erythema. Digital ischaemia mainly affects the toes. Such vascular insufficiency sometimes leads to gangrene and loss of function.
- Stroke.
- Recurrent abortions and fetal growth retardation.
- Hepatic and portal vein thrombosis. The myeloproliferative disorders are the most common causes of hepatic vein thrombosis (Budd–Chiari syndrome).

In addition to thrombotic complications, paradoxically patients with ET, particularly those with a dramatically raised platelet count (over 1500×10^9/L), are at considerably increased risk of bleeding.

Laboratory findings

A raised platelet count, often over 1000×10^9/L, is characteristic of the disorder. The bone marrow shows increased cellularity and plentiful megakaryocytes, but the changes are not specific to the disorder and may occur in reactive states. The diagnosis remains one of exclusion. Certain criteria must be satisfied before the diagnosis can be entertained and these are listed in Table 11.4.

Treatment

Treatment of essential thrombocythaemia is ill defined. There may not be any necessity to treat a young asymptomatic patient and most authorities suggest a risk-based approach. Patients over the age of 60 years, with a platelet count greater than 1500×10^9/L or with a history of thrombosis should be considered for active treatment. The following agents have been used:

- Simple oral chemotherapy with hydroxycarbamide or busulphan for elderly patients.
- α-interferon, which reduces platelet counts but may cause unacceptable side effects such as fatigue, fever, pyrexia and depression. It is the treatment of choice in women of childbearing age due its relative safety in pregnancy.
- Anagrelide, an agent that inhibits megakaryocyte maturation and does not affect the white cell count. It is the preferred treatment in some centres, but can cause vasodilatation, cardiac dysrhythmias and fluid retention.

Antiplatelet drugs such as aspirin can be highly effective in patients at risk of thrombotic episodes. They may be associated with haemorrhage and should not be used in patients with a bleeding tendency.

The survival of patients with essential thrombocythaemia is similar to that of an age-matched population.

12

Bone marrow transplantation

Learning objectives

✓ To understand the use of stem cell infusion following high-dose or myeloablative chemotherapy

✓ To understand the concept of the graft versus leukaemia/lymphoma effect

✓ To understand the nature of graft versus host disease

The idea of rescuing patients by infusing bone marrow after myeloablative chemotherapy or radiotherapy is not a new concept. Animal experiments carried out in the 1950s demonstrated that intravenous infusion of marrow cells could protect against lethal irradiation. Subsequently, successful engraftment was demonstrated in humans.

Bone marrow transplantation may be autologous or allogeneic. In autologous transplantation, the patient's own stem cells are collected following standard chemotherapy treatment. Doses of cytotoxic treatment that ablate the bone marrow are then administered, followed by reinfusion of the collected stem cells. These stem cells repopulate the bone marrow and allow recovery from otherwise supra-lethal doses of chemotherapy or radiotherapy (Table 12.1).

The understanding of the human leucocyte antigen system (HLA) meant that tissue matching between donor and patient was possible and successful bone marrow transplants (BMTs) using matched donors (*allogeneic BMT*) followed in increasing numbers (Figure 12.1). Allogeneic transplantation was initially assumed to be beneficial, because it allowed the administration of doses of cytotoxic treatments that would otherwise have been lethal, totally ablating the native bone marrow, as in autologous transplantation. However, it has since emerged that a critical component of the effectiveness of allogeneic transplantation is the immunologically mediated

Table 12.1 Diseases for which allogeneic and autologous BMT may be considered.

Indications for BMT	Allogeneic BMT	Autologous BMT
Malignant		
Acute leukaemia	+	(+)
Chronic myeloid leukaemia	+	−
Lymphoma (relapsed)	+	+
Myeloma	−	+
Non-malignant		
Aplastic anaemia	+	−
Thalassaemia	+	−
Sickle cell anaemia	+	−

'graft-versus-leukaemia' (GVL) effect, whereby T cells infused as part of the BMT exert a direct antitumour effect. Where there is no immunological difference of donor and recipient, as in identical twin-sibling transplants, there is a higher relapse rate than when a non-twin-sibling matched donor is used; this highlights the importance of the GVL effect in the success of allogeneic transplantation. Indeed, there is increasing reliance on the GVL effect in allogeneic

Haematology Lecture Notes, Ninth edition. C.S.R. Hatton, N.C. Hughes-Jones, D. Hay and D. Keeling. © 2013 John Wiley & Sons, Ltd.
Published 2013 by John Wiley & Sons, Ltd.

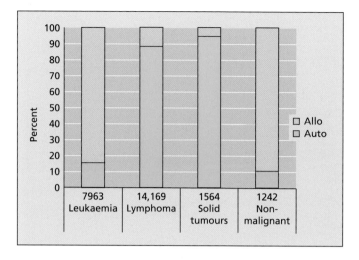

Figure 12.1 The graph shows the number and percentage of allogeneic and autologous stem cell transplants reported in Europe in 2006. The majority of allogeneic stem cell transplants are performed for AML, while the majority of autologous transplants are performed for lymphoma.

transplantation as reduced-intensity conditioning (RIC) regimens become more widely used, with lower doses of cytotoxic treatment.

Allogeneic bone marrow transplantation

The necessary elements for a successful allogeneic BMT include:

- *A source of HLA-matched stem cells.* Stem cells can be collected from an HLA-matched sibling, a matched unrelated donor or in some cases matched umbilical cord blood. The chance of any sibling being a match is one in four, whereas the chance of a volunteer being a match is closer to one in 100 000. Most developed countries have registers of donors against which a patient's HLA type can be matched (Figure 12.2).
- *Immunosuppression* (chemotherapy and radiotherapy) prior to marrow infusion to allow engraftment.
- *Continuing immunosuppression* after infusion to prevent graft-versus-host disease (GVHD).

The process of allogeneic bone marrow transplantation involves:

- *High-dose chemotherapy either with or without total body radiotherapy*: This is used to eradicate the neoplastic cells and to allow engraftment of the donor marrow.
- *Infusion of bone marrow or peripheral blood stem cells*: These are collected directly from the bone marrow of the donor, or by leucopheresis of a donor who has been primed by growth factors such as granulocyte or granulocyte macrophage colony-stimulating factor (G-CSF, GM-CSF).
- *Supportive care*: Following high-dose therapy there is inevitably a period of profound marrow suppression, which typically lasts two to three weeks until the newly infused marrow engrafts. Red cells, platelets and antibiotics are essential to supportive care. Severe mucositis and gastroenteritis often develop and, consequently, many patients require parenteral nutrition during this time.
- *Prevention of GVHD*: A number of immunosuppressive drugs are used to control the immune component (mainly T cells) of the donor-derived engrafted marrow. Ciclosporin is the mainstay of this treatment, but other drugs such as methotrexate and prednisolone are frequently used.

Complications of allogeneic BMT

The principal complication of allogeneic BMT is infection. The severe neutropenia that follows high-dose chemotherapy is frequently complicated by Gram-negative infection. Fungal (*Aspergillus* and *Candida* species) and viral (herpes viruses) infections are also found after allogeneic BMT. The use of steroids to control GVHD further increases the risk of fungal infection.

Cytomegalovirus

Cytomegalovirus (CMV) is a cause of morbidity and mortality in BMT patients. Patients may acquire active CMV infection due to the use of seropositive

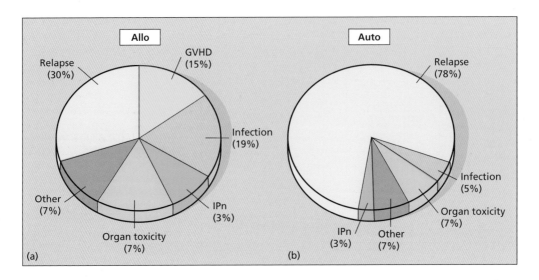

Figure 12.2 Causes of death after transplants done in 1996–2000. *Notes*: GVHD – graft versus host disease; Ipn – interstitial pneumonitis.

marrow donors, seropositive blood products or the reactivation of latent CMV infection in seropositive patients.

Infection and organ damage are related to viral load, which can be detected in the blood by the polymerase chain reaction (PCR). Interstitial pneumonitis is a serious complication of CMV infection, but other organs may be affected, notably the gastrointestinal tract. The use of CMV seronegative blood products in patients who are not already infected helps to reduce the chance of infection. Prophylactic aciclovir and the use of ganciclovir for treatment have reduced the morbidity and mortality from CMV.

Graft-versus-host disease

GVHD results from the reaction of donor T cells against the recipient's tissues; the disorder may be acute or chronic. Prophylactic ciclosporin, a T-cell inhibitor, considerably reduces the incidence and severity of GVHD and is given continuously throughout the immediate post-transplant period. Other drugs such as methotrexate and mycophenolate may be used as alternatives, or in addition to ciclosporin, to prevent GVHD.

Acute GVHD

This may occur during the first 100 days after BMT and chiefly affects the skin, gastrointestinal tract and liver. Skin involvement varies from a mild maculopapular rash to severe desquamation. Gastrointestinal involvement may involve the upper or lower tract.

Symptoms include nausea, vomiting or severe watery diarrhoea. Biopsy is usually required to confirm the diagnosis.

T-cell depletion of the donor marrow reduces the risk of GVHD, and some centres routinely deplete donor marrow this way. T-cell depletion is, however, associated with a higher risk of relapse due to a reduction in the graft-versus-leukaemia effect (GVL; see below). Once established, acute GVHD is a serious disorder with a high mortality. Treatment with high-dose steroids can help, but many patients with severe GVHD die of infection.

Chronic GVHD

Chronic GVHD is a serious complication of BMT occurring after 100 days in approximately 30–40% of patients. The main manifestations are dry eyes, skin changes, chronic liver disease, weight loss and increased risk of infection. The prognosis is poor.

Graft-versus-leukaemia/lymphoma effect

In addition to producing GVHD, the lymphocytes from the graft are also thought to exert an immune effect against the recipient's tumour cells. This is the graft-versus-leukaemia/lymphoma effect (GVL). Patients receiving a BMT for chronic myeloid leukaemia (CML) often have molecular evidence of persistent leukaemia (the presence of the Philadelphia chromosome) in the immediate post-transplant period, although this disappears later, but T-cell depletion of the donor marrow is associated with a higher risk of relapse. This implies that the T cells infused with the donor stem cells are active in eradicating the underlying disease over a period of time. In the event of relapse, the infusion of lymphocytes from the original graft donor (donor lymphocyte infusion, or DLI) has been shown to have a powerful antitumour effect and may induce a further remission, at the cost of increased GVHD.

While the phenomena of GVHD and GVL appear to be intimately related, the exact nature of the underlying molecular targets remains unknown. It may be that minor histocompatibility antigens are important, but evidence suggests that the explanation is more complex than this. GVHD and GVL are not necessarily produced by the same mechanisms: it is one of the key aims of research in this field to try to separate them, to harness the benefits of GVL, while avoiding the severe morbidity of GVHD. The understanding of the process of GVL should provide a powerful tool to eradicate malignant disease.

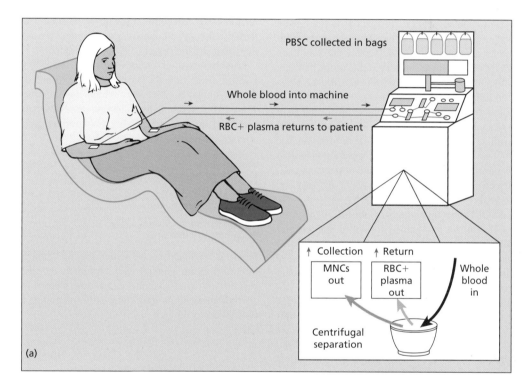

(a)

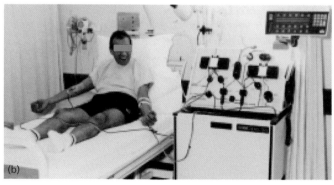

(b)

Figure 12.3 Diagram showing the collection of peripheral blood stem cells using a COBE spectra apheresis machine.
Notes: MNC – mononuclear cell; PBSC – peripheral blood stem cell; RBC – red blood cell.

Mini-allograft or RIC transplant

Reduced intensity conditioning (RIC) allogeneic transplant relies almost entirely on engrafted donor immune cells to eradicate disease – graft-versus-leukaemia/lymphoma effect (GVL; see above). The technique is not dependent on high-dose chemotherapy or total body irradiation to ablate malignant cells, but, rather, uses lower doses of 'conditioning' therapy sufficient to allow the tissue-compatible donor stem cells to engraft. The patient is then given ciclosporin or an equivalent T-cell suppressant drug to limit the development of GVHD following donor cell engraftment. There is a balance to be struck between the benefits of GVL and the harmful effects of GVHD.

The lower dose of chemotherapy or radiotherapy reduces the toxicity and therefore the mortality of the procedure. The mini-allogeneic transplant or RIC transplant has particular relevance to an older age group, since full allogeneic transplantation is limited to patients under 45–50 years of age, whereas the RIC transplant may be tolerated by patients up to the age of 65 years of age.

Extremely encouraging results for RIC allografting are emerging for low-grade lymphoproliferative and myeloproliferative disorders, and there is evidence to suggest that the immune response is capable of controlling and destroying more aggressive disorders such as acute leukaemia.

Although more readily tolerated than full allografting, the mortality of this procedure is still in the order of between 10% and 20% in most of the reported series; the morbidity and mortality of GVHD remain a significant problem.

Autologous bone marrow transplantation (high-dose therapy)

In autologous BMT, the patient's own marrow stem cells are used to reconstitute the bone marrow after intensive chemotherapy with or without radiotherapy. There is therefore no requirement for tissue matching and the risk of GVHD is eliminated.

Chemotherapy or radiotherapy acts by killing a fraction of the tumour. Dose is, however, limited by the myeloablative effects of very high-dose treatment. This can be overcome by collecting stem cells before high-dose therapy and infusing them into the patient after intensive conditioning therapy.

There are four phases of high-dose therapy:

1 Marrow harvest/peripheral blood stem cell harvest (Figure 12.3).
2 Conditioning therapy.
3 Reinfusion of the stem cells.
4 Supportive therapy.

Stem cells can be collected either directly by marrow puncture under general anaesthesia or by apheresis. In both cases patients need to be primed with chemotherapy and granulocyte-stimulating factor (G-CSF).

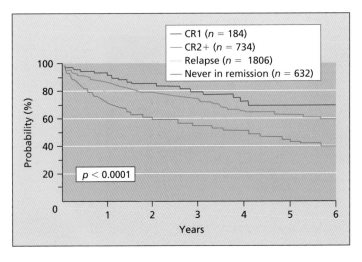

Figure 12.4 The probability of survival after autotransplants for Hodgkin lymphoma.
Note: CR – complete remission.

A serious disadvantage of autologous BMT is the potential for reinfusing malignant cells. Various purging strategies have been tried in an effort to reduce this risk, but none has so far been shown to affect outcome positively.

Supportive therapy is very similar to the care given after any intensive chemotherapy. Blood products – red cells and platelet concentrates – together with antibiotics and nutritional support are the fundamentals of therapy at this stage. Most patients will engraft after two to three weeks, and some centres use G-CSF or GM-CSF to limit the duration of neutropenia.

The principal indications for this type of procedure include relapsed Hodgkin lymphoma (Figure 12.4) and non-Hodgkin lymphoma and myeloma in younger patients.

13

Aplastic anaemia and pure red cell aplasia

Learning objectives

✓ To know the aetiology of acquired aplastic anaemia, including the drugs that have been most commonly reported to cause this syndrome

✓ To know the clinical and laboratory features, the natural history and the principles of treatment of acquired aplastic anaemia

✓ To understand the difference between aplastic anaemia and pure red cell aplasia

Aplastic anaemia

Aplastic anaemia is a disorder characterized by pancytopenia (i.e. a reduction in the number of red cells, neutrophils and platelets in the peripheral blood), a marked decrease in the amount of haemopoietic tissue in the bone marrow (i.e. marrow aplasia or hypoplasia) and the absence of evidence of involvement of the marrow by diseases such as leukaemia, myeloma or carcinoma. The causes of aplastic anaemia are summarized in Table 13.1.

Acquired aplastic anaemia

This is an uncommon disease, the prevalence in Europe being between 1 and 3 per 100 000 people. It affects all ages with two peaks, one in adolescents and young adults and the other in people over the age of 60 years.

Aetiology

In about half of cases no aetiological factors can be identified; such patients are described as having idiopathic acquired aplastic anaemia. In the others, the aplasia is associated with exposure to certain drugs or chemicals, ionizing radiation or certain viruses.

Most cases of secondary aplastic anaemia result from an idiosyncratic reaction to the use of antirheumatic drugs (e.g. phenylbutazone, indomethacin, ibuprofen or sodium aurothiomalate), chloramphenicol, trimethoprim-sulphamethoxazole (cotrimoxazole) or organic arsenicals. Many other drugs have been less commonly implicated and these include anticonvulsants (phenytoin, carbamazepine), antithyroid drugs (carbimazole, propylthiouracil), mepacrine and chlorpromazine. Some drugs regularly cause aplastic anaemia if given in sufficiently large doses: these include alkylating agents (e.g. busulphan, melphalan

Table 13.1 **Causes of aplastic anaemia.**

Congenital

Fanconi anaemia

Acquired

Idiopathic

Drugs and chemicals

    Dose-dependent: Cytotoxic drugs, benzene

    Idiosyncratic: Chloramphenicol, non-steroidal anti-inflammatory drugs

Radiation

Viruses: Hepatitis non-A, non-B, non-C, Epstein–Barr virus

Paroxysmal nocturnal haemoglobinuria

Haematology Lecture Notes, Ninth edition. C.S.R. Hatton, N.C. Hughes-Jones, D. Hay and D. Keeling. © 2013 John Wiley & Sons, Ltd. Published 2013 by John Wiley & Sons, Ltd.

Pathophysiology

The pancytopenia and marrow aplasia appear to be the consequence of damage to the multipotent haemopoietic stem cells, which impairs their self-renewal (pp. 1–2) and causes stem cell depletion. This damage may be caused by some drugs or viruses or by cell-mediated immunological mechanisms. The possibility that stromal (microenvironmental) cell damage may be the primary defect has also been considered, but this is unlikely to be true in most cases because of the success of stem cell transplantation.

Clinical features

Both idiopathic and secondary aplastic anaemia occur at all ages. The onset is often insidious but may be acute. Symptoms include:

- lassitude, weakness and shortness of breath due to anaemia
- haemorrhagic manifestations resulting from the thrombocytopenia
- fever and recurrent infections as a consequence of neutropenia.

Haemorrhagic manifestations include epistaxis, bleeding from the gums, menorrhagia, bleeding into the gastrointestinal and urinary tracts, and ecchymoses and petechiae. The severity of the symptoms is variable and depends on the severity of the cytopenias. In patients with severe neutropenia and thrombocytopenia, fulminating infections (e.g. pneumonia) and cerebral haemorrhage are common causes of death. In secondary aplastic anaemia, symptoms may appear several weeks or months, or occasionally one or more years, after discontinuation of exposure to the causative drug or chemical. Splenomegaly is rare in aplastic anaemia, and if the spleen is palpable alternative diagnoses should be explored.

Haematological findings

There is a normochromic or macrocytic anaemia associated with a low absolute reticulocyte count. The platelet count is often below 100×10^9/L, and may be very low. Neutropenia and monocytopenia are usually found at some stage of the disease. Some patients also have a reduced absolute lymphocyte count. There is a marked increase in serum and urinary erythropoietin levels.

Markedly hypocellular marrow fragments are usually found in marrow smears, most of the volume of the marrow fragments being made up of fat cells (Figure 13.1). Haemopoietic cells of all types, including megakaryocytes, are decreased or absent, and in

and cyclophosphamide), antipurines, antipyrimidines and antifolates. Benzene is an example of an industrial chemical that often produces aplastic anaemia if inhaled in a sufficient dose; kerosene, carbon tetrachloride and certain insecticides, such as DDT and chlordane, can also cause aplasia of the marrow.

Aplastic anaemia may develop after a single large dose of whole-body irradiation (e.g. during atomic bomb explosions or radiation accidents). It was also seen in the past following repeated radiotherapy to the spine in patients with ankylosing spondylitis.

Severe aplastic anaemia, usually with a poor prognosis, may rarely develop in children and young adults about 10 weeks after an episode of acute non-A, non-B and non-C hepatitis. Marrow aplasia is also a rare complication of Epstein–Barr virus infection.

The T-lymphocytes of some patients with acquired aplastic anaemia inhibit the *in vitro* growth of haemopoietic colonies from autologous and allogeneic bone marrow. This finding, together with the response of about 50% of patients to antilymphocyte globulin, indicates that autoimmune mechanisms are involved in at least the persistence of the aplasia, if not its initiation, in a number of cases.

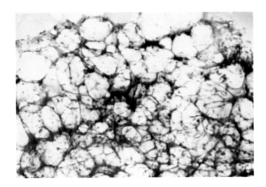

Figure 13.1 Markedly hypocellular marrow fragment from a case of aplastic anaemia. There are only a few residual haemopoietic cells, most of the fragments consisting of fat cells.

Table 13.2 **Causes of pancytopenia.**
Mainly due to a failure of production of cells
Bone marrow infiltration: leukaemia, myeloma, carcinoma, myelofibrosis, lipid storage disorders, marble bone disease
Severe vitamin B12 or folate deficiency
Myelodysplastic syndromes
HIV infection
Aplastic or hypoplastic anaemia
Mainly due to an increased peripheral destruction of cells
Splenomegaly
Overwhelming infection
Systemic lupus erythematosus (SLE)
Paroxysmal nocturnal haemoglobinuria*
Note: * In some cases, there is also impaired production of cells due to hypoplasia of the marrow.

severe aplastic anaemia the majority of the cells seen are plasma cells, lymphocytes and macrophages. Residual erythropoietic cells are morphologically abnormal. Although the marrow is generally hypocellular, it contains some foci of normal or even increased cellularity. Thus, even in patients with severe aplastic anaemia, marrow aspiration may occasionally yield normocellular or hypercellular fragments. In order to obtain a reliable estimate of marrow cellularity, it is essential to examine histological sections of a trephine biopsy of the iliac crest (Figure 13.2). This not only provides a larger volume of marrow for study than a single marrow aspirate, but also permits the detection of foci of leukaemia cells, myeloma cells or carcinoma cells, if present.

Some patients with acquired aplastic anaemia develop the red cell defect seen in paroxysmal nocturnal

haemoglobinuria (p. 34), without or with haemoglobinuria. Occasionally patients develop a terminal acute leukaemia.

Diagnosis

Other causes of pancytopenia (particularly leukaemia) should be considered and excluded before a diagnosis of aplastic anaemia is made. The causes of pancytopenia are summarized in Table 13.2.

Prognosis

Patients with both idiopathic and secondary acquired aplastic anaemia show a highly variable clinical course. About 15% of patients have a severe illness from the outset and die within 3 months of diagnosis. Overall, as many as 50% of cases die within 15 months of diagnosis and 70% within 5 years. Only about 10% make a complete haematological recovery. If a patient survives for longer than 18 months, there is a reasonable chance of prolonged survival and complete recovery. Poor prognostic features include a platelet count less than 20×10^9/L, a neutrophil count below 0.2×10^9/L, a reticulocyte count under 10×10^9/L and marked hypocellularity of the marrow.

Treatment

If a causative drug or chemical is identified, exposure to this agent should be immediately stopped. Supportive therapy including red cell transfusions and

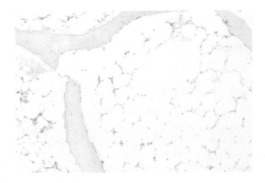

Figure 13.2 Section of a trephine biopsy of the bone marrow from a patient with aplastic anaemia showing marked hypocellularity (haemotoxylin and eosin).

antibiotics should be administered when necessary; the extent of supportive therapy required depends on the degree of cytopenia. Platelet transfusions are only indicated if haemorrhage becomes a serious problem, as repeated platelet transfusions lead to alloimmunization and a reduction of the efficacy of subsequent platelet transfusions.

Bone marrow transplantation is indicated at diagnosis for patients under 40 years with severe aplastic anaemia (i.e. showing the poor prognostic features mentioned above), particularly if an HLA-compatible sibling donor is available. Long-term survival is seen in 60–80% of cases; graft rejection is more of a problem in aplastic anaemia than in other conditions. Patients who are not transplanted may benefit from treatment with antithymocyte globulin (ATG), cyclosporin A, methylprednisolone, androgens or the anabolic steroid oxymetholone (which causes less virilization of females than androgens). Combined immunosuppressive regimens have been shown to be more effective than single-agent therapy. The addition of granulocyte colony-stimulating factor (G-CSF) has also produced encouraging results. The overall survival for patients with severe aplastic anaemia has improved considerably and is now greater than 70% at five years.

Pure red cell aplasia

Rarely, aplasia or severe hypoplasia affects only the erythropoietic cells. Patients with this abnormality have anaemia and reticulocytopenia together with normal white cell and platelet counts.

The causes of pure red cell aplasia are listed in Table 13.3. In the rare congenital form – Diamond Blackfan anaemia – anaemia usually develops in infancy and is associated with various congenital malformations, including craniofacial abnormalities and those of the thumb and upper limbs. About a quarter of cases have a mutation in the ribosome protein S19 gene.

Acquired pure red cell aplasia may present as an acute self-limiting condition (e.g. when it follows a parvovirus B19 infection) or as a chronic disorder. The reticulocytopenia that follows parvovirus B19 infection in normal individuals does not significantly lower the haemoglobin level because red cells survive for such a long time. In patients with haemolytic anaemia when red cell survival is reduced (e.g. sickle cell anaemia), parvovirus infection leads to severe anaemia, which may be life threatening. Patients with

Table 13.3 Causes of pure red cell aplasia.

Congenital

Diamond–Blackfan syndrome (congenital erythroblastopenia or erythrogenesis imperfecta)

Acquired

Idiopathic

Viral infections: Parvovirus B19 (p. 28), Epstein–Barr virus, hepatitis

Drugs and chemicals: Phenytoin sodium, azathioprine, erythropoietin, benzene

Thymic tumours

Lymphoid malignancies: Chronic lymphocytic leukaemia, lymphoma

Other malignant diseases: Carcinoma of the bronchus, breast, stomach and thyroid

Autoimmune disorders: SLE, rheumatoid arthritis

this complication present with severe pallor, white sclera (normally yellow in chronic haemolysis) and other symptoms of severe anaemia.

Immunological mechanisms, both cellular and humoral, may underlie the aplasia in some patients with chronic pure red cell aplasia (e.g. those with thymoma, chronic lymphocytic leukaemia or autoimmune disorders). A small number of patients with renal failure who have been given subcutaneous recombinant human erythropoietin have developed red cell aplasia. The mechanism is thought to reflect the development of neutralizing anti-erythropoietin antibodies.

Some patients with chronic pure red cell aplasia respond to immunosuppressive drugs such as corticosteroids, azathioprine, cyclophosphamide, cyclosporin A or antithymocyte globulin. Patients with persistent parvovirus infection respond to intravenous injections of immunoglobulin.

Box 13.2 Parvovirus B19

The parvovirus B19 enters erythroid progenitor cells (by binding to the P blood group antigen), replicates within these cells and damages them. In most patients the infection and erythroblastopenia are transient, but in patients with certain congenital or acquired immunological disorders, there is persistence of the infection and of the red cell aplasia.

14

Haemostasis, abnormal bleeding and anticoagulant therapy

Learning objectives

✓ To know the function of platelets and the relationship between the platelet count in peripheral blood and the extent of abnormal bleeding

✓ To know about the diseases associated with (i) a failure of platelet production and (ii) a shortened platelet lifespan, especially immune thrombocytopenic purpura (ITP)

✓ To know the main sequence of events in the coagulation pathways

✓ To understand normal fibrinolysis and the principles of fibrinolytic therapy

✓ To know the principles underlying the prothrombin time (PT), activated partial thromboplastin time (APTT) and thrombin time (TT)

✓ To know the principles of investigation of a patient suspected of having a haemostatic defect

✓ To know the mode of inheritance, clinical presentation, method of diagnosis and principles of treatment of haemophilia A (factor FVIII deficiency), haemophilia B (factor IX deficiency) and von Willebrand disease (VWD)

✓ To know the effects of vitamin K deficiency and liver disease on the clotting mechanisms

✓ To know the alterations in the haemostatic and fibrinolytic mechanisms associated with disseminated intravascular coagulation (DIC) and the causes of DIC

✓ To understand the principles of anticoagulant therapy with unfractionated heparin, low molecular weight heparin and warfarin and to know about the laboratory control of such therapy

✓ To be aware of the natural anticoagulant mechanisms in blood and some of the prothrombotic states (thrombophilia)

Haematology Lecture Notes, Ninth edition. C.S.R. Hatton, N.C. Hughes-Jones, D. Hay and D. Keeling. © 2013 John Wiley & Sons, Ltd.
Published 2013 by John Wiley & Sons, Ltd.

Normal haemostasis

The cessation of bleeding following trauma to blood vessels results from three processes: (i) the contraction of vessel walls; (ii) the formation of a platelet plug at the site of the break in the vessel wall; and (iii) the formation of a fibrin clot. The clot forms within and around the platelet aggregates and results in a firm haemostatic plug. The relative importance of these three processes probably varies according to the size of the vessels involved. Thus, in bleeding from a minor wound, the formation of a haemostatic plug is probably sufficient in itself, whereas in larger vessels, contraction of the vessel walls also plays a part in haemostasis. The initial plug is formed almost entirely of platelets, but this is friable and is subsequently stabilized by fibrin formation.

Classification of haemostatic defects

The action of platelets and the clotting mechanism are closely intertwined in the prevention of bleeding. However, it is convenient to consider that abnormalities in haemostasis resulting in bleeding arise from defects in one of three processes:

1 Thrombocytopenia (a low platelet count) (the commonest cause).
2 Abnormal platelet function.
3 A defect in the clotting mechanism (the second commonest cause).

A clinical distinction can frequently be made between bleeding due to clotting defects and bleeding due to a diminished number of platelets. Patients with clotting defects usually present with bleeding into deep tissues; that is, muscles or joints. Patients with a deficiency of platelets usually present with mucocutaneous bleeding; that is, bleeding into the skin and from the epithelial surfaces of the nose, uterus and other organs. Haemorrhages into the skin include petechiae, which are less than 1 mm in diameter (Figure 14.1), and ecchymoses, which are larger than petechiae and vary considerably in size (Figure 14.2). A further useful clinical distinction is that bleeding usually persists from the time of injury in the case of platelet deficiency, since platelet numbers are inadequate to form a good platelet plug, whereas in clotting defects the initial bleeding may cease in normal time as platelet plugs are readily formed, but as a

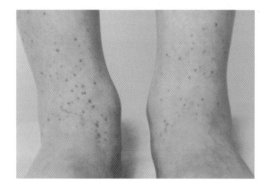

Figure 14.1 Multiple pin-point haemorrhages (petechiae) on the legs of a patient with idiopathic thrombocytopenic purpura (ITP).

consequence of the failure to form an adequate clot the platelet plug is not stabilized by fibrin formation and subsequently disintegrates, resulting in a delayed onset of prolonged bleeding. The clinical distinction is by no means complete, as deep-seated haemorrhage is sometimes found in platelet deficiency and, on the other hand, superficial bleeding may occur in clotting defects.

Petechial haemorrhages and ecchymoses and bleeding from other sites may occur when the number of platelets falls below 50×10^9/L. At levels between 20 and 50×10^9/L, petechiae, ecchymoses and nose bleeds are the commonest symptoms, but below 20×10^9/L, gross haemorrhage (melaena, haematemesis, haematuria) becomes increasingly common. However, there is a great deal of variation in the relationship between the platelet count and haemorrhage in individual patients.

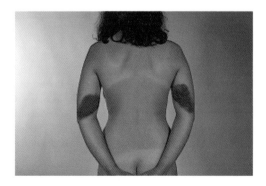

Figure 14.2 Large ecchymoses on both the upper arms of a woman with ITP.

Platelets

Morphology and lifespan

Platelets are discoid, non-nucleated, granule-containing cells (2–3 μm in diameter) that are formed in the bone marrow by the fragmentation of megakaryocyte cytoplasm. Their concentration in normal blood is $150–450 \times 10^9/L$.

The plasma membrane of a platelet contains glycoproteins (GPs) that are important in the interaction of platelets with subendothelial connective tissue and other platelets. These include GP Ia and VI, which bind to collagen; GP Ib, which binds to von Willebrand factor (VWF); and GP IIb/IIIa, which binds to fibrinogen. The platelet membrane is extensively invaginated to form a surface-connected canalicular system through which the contents of platelet granules are released. Another intracellular membrane system known as the dense tubular system is rich in calcium, phospholipid-bound arachidonic acid, phospholipase A_2 (which mobilizes arachidonic acid), cyclo-oxygenase and thromboxane synthase, and is the main site of prostaglandin and thromboxane synthesis. The platelet also contains contractile microfilaments, an equatorial band of microtubules involved in maintaining its normal discoid shape and two main types of ultrastructurally identifiable granules. The α-granules, which are the most numerous, contain platelet factor 4 (heparin-neutralizing factor), platelet-derived growth factor (which stimulates mitosis in vascular smooth muscle cells), VWF and fibrinogen. The contents of the dense granules (δ-granules) include adenosine triphosphate (ATP), adenosine disphosphate (ADP), 5-hydroxytryptamine (which causes vasoconstriction) and calcium.

The lifespan of the platelet has been determined by labelling platelets *in vitro* with radioactive chromium (^{51}Cr) and studying their fate after reinjection into the circulation; it is of the order of 10 days.

Physiology

The main function of platelets is the formation of a haemostatic plug at sites of damage to vascular endothelium. First the platelets adhere to exposed subendothelial collagen (via GP Ia and VI) and VWF (via GpIb). Within 1–2 s of adhesion, platelets change their shape from a disc to a more rounded form with spicules that encourage platelet–platelet interaction. and they also release the contents of their granules (platelet release reaction), the most important content of which is ADP. The platelets are also stimulated

to produce the prostaglandin, thromboxane A_2 from arachidonic acid derived from the cell membrane. The release of ADP and thromboxane A_2 causes an interaction of other platelets with the adherent platelets and with each other (secondary platelet aggregation), thus leading to the formation of a platelet plug (primary haemostasis). On the surface of activated platelets, GP IIb/IIIa undergoes a conformational change to provide binding sites for fibrinogen, which plays a role in linking platelets together to form aggregates. Anionic platelet membrane phospholipids are also exteriorized, providing a procoagulant surface on which important reactions of the coagulation pathway take place. Prostacyclin released by endothelial and vascular smooth muscle cells inhibits platelet aggregation and may thus limit the extent of the platelet plug. Whereas thromboxane A_2 is a potent vasoconstrictor, prostacyclin is a powerful vasodilator.

At the site of injury, tissue factor (TF) is expressed and the TF–VIIa complex initiates the formation of a fibrin clot within and around the platelet plug (secondary haemostasis). The anionic phospholipids exposed on the surface of aggregated platelets allow binding of the vitamin K-dependent proteins (factors II, IX and X) and the cofactors V and VIII, thus considerably enhancing the speed of the clotting reaction on and around the platelet surface. Platelets are also responsible for the contraction of the fibrin clot once it has been formed.

Tests of platelet function

Bleeding time

This used to be a commonly performed test. The bleeding time is estimated by making small wounds in the skin of the forearm after applying a blood pressure cuff to the upper arm and inflating it to 40mmHg; the average time that elapses until bleeding ceases is then measured. The test has poor sensitivity and poor specificity for detecting abnormalities of platelet function, is a poor predictor of bleeding from surgery and invasive procedures and has largely been abandoned.

PFA-100

The bleeding time has largely been replaced by an *in vitro* estimation of primary haemostasis using a machine called a PFA-100. Platelets are passed through a membrane coated with collagen and either ADP or epinephrine, and the time taken for flow to cease measured. Some use this test to rule out a platelet defect when the pre-test probability is low, but it can be normal in some platelet disorders and platelet aggregation studies are required if a platelet defect is a likely possibility, even if PFA closure times are normal.

Platelet aggregation studies

A large number of *in vitro* tests of platelet function have been described, but the most common is light transmission aggregometry, whereby the aggregation of platelets is studied following the addition of substances such as ADP, epinephrine, arachidonate, collagen and ristocetin to platelet-rich plasma. Aggregation causes an increase in the light transmitted through the sample and the test is performed using special equipment capable of continuously recording light transmission.

Thrombocytopenic and non-thrombocytopenic purpura

'Purpura' is the collective term for bleeding into the skin or mucous membranes. Patients with purpura can be separated into those with low platelet counts (thrombocytopenic) and those with normal platelet counts (non-thrombocytopenic). The non-thrombocytopenic group can be subdivided into those patients who have qualitative platelet defects and a group who have vascular abnormalities. The latter is a miscellaneous group and contains congenital disorders such as hereditary haemorrhagic telangiectasia (Figure 14.3) and the Ehlers–Danlos syndrome, and acquired diseases such as Henoch–Schönlein purpura (a vasculitis) and scurvy.

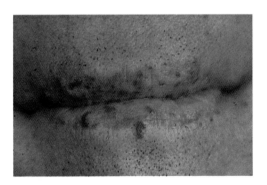

Figure 14.3 Vascular malformations (reddish purple) on the lips of a patient with hereditary haemorrhagic telangiectasia; such lesions are found throughout the body and increase in number with advancing age. This rare condition is inherited as an autosomal dominant characteristic and may lead to recurrent gastrointestinal haemorrhage and chronic iron deficiency anaemia.

Causes of thrombocytopenia

The mechanisms leading to thrombocytopenia are:

- A failure of platelet production by the megakaryocytes.
- A shortened lifespan of the platelets.
- Increased pooling of platelets in an enlarged spleen.

The distinction between the first two of these possibilities can be made by assessing the number of megakaryocytes in a marrow aspirate or trephine biopsy of the marrow.

The causes of thrombocytopenia are given in Table 14.1.

Table 14.1 Some causes of thrombocytopenia.

Failure of platelet production

  Aplastic anaemia

  Drugs

  Viruses

  Myelodysplasia

  Paroxysmal nocturnal haemoglobinuria

  Bone marrow infiltration (carcinoma, leukaemia, lymphoma, myeloma, myelofibrosis, storage diseases including Gaucher's disease, osteopetrosis)

  Megaloblastic anaemia due to B12 or folate deficiency

  Hereditary thrombocytopenia (e.g. thrombocytopenia with absent radii, grey platelet syndrome, Bernard–Soulier syndrome, Wiskott–Aldrich syndrome)

Shortened platelet survival

Immune

  Autoimmune (idiopathic) thrombocytopenic purpura

  Secondary autoimmune thrombocytopenic purpura (SLE and other collagen diseases, lymphoma, chronic lymphocytic leukaemia, HIV infection)

  Drugs

  Post-transfusion purpura

  Neonatal alloimmune thrombocytopenia

  Thrombotic thrombocytopenic purpura (most cases)

Non-immune

  Disseminated intravascular coagulation (p. 127)

Increased splenic pooling

Failure of platelet production

If megakaryocytes are few or absent, it may be assumed that platelet production is at fault. The bone marrow smears may also reveal other features that indicate the nature of the disease if evidence has not already been obtained from the peripheral blood. Thus, there may be a generalized aplasia of the bone marrow (aplastic anaemia) or a selective decrease in megakaryocytes caused by certain drugs (e.g. chlorothiazides, tolbutamide), alcoholism and certain viruses (e.g. Epstein–Barr virus, measles, varicella, cytomegalovirus). Another cause of reduced platelet production is marked infiltration of the marrow by malignant cells (e.g. in leukaemia, lymphoma, myeloma and carcinoma) or by fibrous tissue. Reduced platelet production may also occur in patients with normal or increased numbers of megakaryocytes when there is ineffective megakaryocytopoiesis, as in severe vitamin B12 or folate deficiency or in myelodysplastic syndromes.

Shortened platelet survival

If the megakaryocytes in the marrow are numerous, then the thrombocytopenia is usually due to an excessive rate of removal of platelets from the peripheral circulation. In most cases the destruction results from autoantibodies attached to the platelet surface and the disease is termed (auto)immune thrombocytopenic purpura (ITP). Occasionally it is due to intravascular platelet consumption due to DIC or microangiopathic haemolytic anaemia (e.g. thrombotic thrombocytopenic purpura (TTP) or the haemolytic uraemic syndrome).

Immune thrombocytopenic purpura (ITP)

ITP is characterized by petechiae (Figure 14.1), bruising (Figure 14.2), spontaneous bleeding from mucous membranes and a reduction in the platelet count (without neutropenia or, usually, anaemia). The disease presents in both an acute and a chronic form. The pathogenic mechanism was previously thought to be due to IgG autoantibodies that result in a shortened platelet lifespan due to premature destruction in the spleen. It is now accepted that more complex mechanisms in which both impaired platelet production and T cell-mediated effects play a role.

Clinical features

Acute ITP

This is seen at all ages but is most common before the age of 10 years. Two-thirds of patients give a history of a common childhood viral infection (e.g. upper respiratory tract infection, chicken pox, measles) 2–3 weeks preceding the purpura. Platelet counts are often less than $20 \times 10^9/L$. In most patients the disease runs a self-limiting course of 2–4 weeks, but in approximately 20% it becomes chronic; that is, it lasts more than 6 months. The disease is almost always self-limiting when there is a history of preceding infection. The mortality is low, the main danger being intracranial bleeding.

Chronic ITP

This occurs mainly in the age period 15–50 years; it has a higher incidence in women than in men. The chronic form is usually not severe and mortality is low; platelet counts are usually between 20 and $80 \times 10^9/L$. Spontaneous cures are rare and the disease is characterized by relapses and remissions. About one third of patients with chronic ITP have petechiae and ecchymoses as the only presenting signs. The remainder also have bleeding from the following sites in decreasing order of frequency: nose, gums, vagina (menorrhagia) and gastrointestinal and renal tracts. Cerebral haemorrhage occurs in about 3%. As a general rule the spleen is not palpable.

Diagnosis

Children with the appropriate clinical features, acute thrombocytopenia and an otherwise normal blood count (i.e. no evidence of acute leukaemia) may be diagnosed as having acute ITP without bone marrow aspiration. The diagnosis of chronic ITP is also based on clinical features and the exclusion of other causes of thrombocytopenia and may not require marrow aspiration. In ITP, bone marrow megakaryocytes are normal or increased in number (up to four- or eightfold) and increased in size. An absence or reduction of megakaryocytes rules out the disease. A marrow aspiration also serves to exclude other causes of thrombocytopenia, such as aplastic anaemia, leukaemia or marrow infiltration by carcinoma cells, lymphoma cells or myeloma cells. Thrombocytopenia due to drugs must also be excluded.

Treatment

Acute ITP

Over 80% of patients recover without any treatment. Corticosteroids are widely used: they increase the platelet count and so reduce the duration of thrombocytopenia. High doses of intravenous immunoglobulin (Ig) cause a rapid increase in the platelet count and are administered, with or without corticosteroids, to children with severe thrombocytopenia or life-threatening haemorrhage.

Chronic ITP

Treatment is usually not needed in patients with platelet counts above 30–50×10^9/L who have no significant spontaneous bleeding. High-dose corticosteroid therapy increases the platelet count to more than 50×10^9/L and, usually, more than 100×10^9/L in two-thirds of patients with chronic ITP. Adults are often started on prednisolone 60 mg/day and the dosage reduced gradually after a remission is achieved, or after 4 weeks. However, in only a third of patients who initially have a complete remission is the remission long lived.

Splenectomy and a large number of drugs have been used as second-line treatment. About 75% of the patients respond fully to splenectomy, usually within 1 week. However, 10–15% of complete responders will relapse after an interval.

Azathioprine, cyclophosphamide, danazol, dapsone, cyclosporine A, mycophenolate mofetil and rituximab have all been used, particularly in patients who fail to respond to splenectomy.

High dose of intravenous Ig (e.g. 1 g/kg/day for 2 days) has also been found to increase the platelet count to greater than 50×10^9/L in 80% of patients with chronic ITP and to normal values in more than 50%. However, the increase is usually transient; the platelet count returns to pretreatment levels in 2–6 weeks. Ig probably acts by interfering with platelet destruction by inhibiting the binding of the Fc portion of the IgG antibodies on the platelet surface to Fc receptors on macrophages. Anti-D Ig (in patients who are Rhesus D+) is thought to work in the same way.

Most recently, thrombopoietin-receptor agonists (romiplostin and eltrombopag) have been shown to be effective in clinical trials.

Secondary autoimmune thrombocytopenic purpura

An autoimmune thrombocytopenia may precede other manifestations of SLE by several years and may complicate the course of SLE, other autoimmune disorders, lymphoma and chronic lymphocytic leukaemia. Patients infected with the human immunodeficiency virus (HIV) may develop either autoimmune thrombocytopenia or immune thrombocytopenia (caused by immune complexes) long before developing other characteristic features.

Drug-induced immune thrombocytopenia

Certain drugs such as heparin, gold salts, quinine, quinidine, sulphonamides or penicillin cause a short-ening of platelet lifespan in a small proportion of recipients by an immunological mechanism. Heparin induced thrombocytopenia (HIT) is particularly important. Antibodies form against the heparin:platelet factor 4 (PF4) complex and then bind to the platelet FcγR, causing platelet activation, thrombocytopenia and in some instances seemingly paradoxical thrombosis.

Other immune thrombocytopenias

In the rare condition known as post-transfusion purpura, severe thrombocytopenia develops 5–8 days after a transfusion, as a result of the destruction of the recipient's platelets. Platelet-specific alloantibodies are present in the serum, but the explanation for the destruction of the patient's own platelets is unclear.

Transient but potentially serious neonatal alloimmune thrombocytopenia may occur in babies of healthy mothers. The mother forms IgG alloantibodies against a fetal platelet-specific antigen lacking in the mother's platelets and inherited from the father; these antibodies cross the placenta and damage fetal platelets (analogous to haemolytic disease of the newborn).

Thrombotic thrombocytopenic purpura (TTP)

In healthy individuals a VWF-cleaving protease (ADAMTS 13) cleaves the Tyr 842-Met 843 peptide bond in VWF to produce the characteristic multimer profile. In the absence of the protease, ultra-large VWF multimers are released that lead to platelet aggregation and the disease known as 'thrombotic thrombocytopenic purpura' (TTP). Familial relapsing TTP is due to the autosomal recessive inheritance of a deficiency of the protease. Sporadic TTP is due to an IgG autoantibody against the protease. This is a serious illness characterized by widespread arteriolar platelet thrombi leading to fragmentation of red cells, thrombocytopenia, neurological symptoms and renal impairment. It is an important diagnosis to make because the untreated mortality is 90%, which can be reduced with the prompt delivery of plasma exchange. The haemolytic uraemic syndrome is an apparently similar disorder affecting infants, young children and the elderly in which the arteriolar thrombi are predominantly formed in the kidneys; in some patients, the disease follows a bout of diarrhoea caused by verotoxin-producing *Escherichia coli* or shiga toxin-producing *Shigella dysenteriae*. It is not due to a deficiency of ADAMTS 13 and does not respond to plasma exchange.

Increased splenic pooling

A normal spleen contains within its microcirculation about 30% of all the blood platelets; the platelets in the splenic pool exchange freely with those in the general circulation. The splenic platelet pool increases with increasing splenic size, so that in patients with moderate to massive splenomegaly it may account for 50–90% of all blood platelets, thus causing thrombocytopenia. Another factor contributing to the thrombocytopenia in patients with splenomegaly is an increase in plasma volume.

Abnormalities of platelet function

Acquired

An acquired defect of platelet function is found after ingestion of aspirin and other antiplatelet drugs. Aspirin acts by irreversibly acetylating cyclo-oxygenase and this inhibits thromboxane A_2 synthesis, with a subsequent reduction in platelet aggregation. The effect of a single dose of aspirin can be detected for 1 week (i.e. until most of the platelets present at the time of taking the aspirin have been replaced by newly formed platelets). Clopidogrel acts by irreversibly blocking the ADP receptor (P2Y12) on the platelet cell membrane.

Other causes of an acquired abnormality of platelet function include chronic myeloproliferative disorders, myelodysplastic syndromes, paraproteinaemias (e.g. myeloma or Waldenström's macroglobulinaemia) and uraemia.

Inherited

Glanzmann's disease

This is a rare but severe platelet disorder caused by a lack of glycoprotein IIb/IIIa receptors. Inheritance is autosomal recessive and platelets are normal in morphology and number.

Bernard-Soulier disease

This is a platelet disorder caused by a lack of glycoprotein Ib receptors. Inheritance is autosomal recessive. Platelets are larger than normal and usually the platelet count is reduced.

Storage pool diseases

These are inherited conditions resulting in defective platelet granules. In the more common δ-storage pool disease there is a deficiency of dense granules. It can occur alone or in the patients with Hermansky-Pudlak syndrome, when it is combined with albinism and ocular defects.

Platelet transfusions

It is often possible to raise the platelet count temporarily by platelet transfusions. The main indication for platelet transfusion is severe haemorrhage caused by (i) thrombocytopenia due to diminished platelet production or DIC; or (ii) abnormal platelet function. Transfusion may also be indicated in a patient with thrombocytopenia or defective platelet function prior to surgery. Another indication for platelet transfusion is thrombocytopenia (platelets $<50 \times 10^9$/L) in patients receiving massive blood transfusions; blood stored for 48 hours has virtually no viable platelets. When thrombocytopenia results from excess destruction caused by platelet antibodies, the response to transfusion is poor. Platelets are transfused as platelet concentrates and should be given within five days of withdrawal from the donor. In order to prevent *spontaneous* haemorrhage, platelet counts need only be maintained above $10–20 \times 10^9$/L, since severe bleeding is rare above this level.

Normal coagulation mechanism

The mechanisms involved in the clotting cascade were elucidated in the period 1950–70, largely by the work of R.G. MacFarlane and his colleagues. The essential feature of the cascade is the presence of a number of steps activated in sequence. Each step is characterized by the conversion of a zymogen (proenzyme) into an enzyme by the splitting of one or more peptide bonds, which brings about a conformational change in the molecule and reveals the active enzyme site.

The clotting sequence is initiated *in vivo* by tissue factor (TF) exposed on the surface of activated endothelial cells and leucocytes and on most extravascular cells in an area of tissue damage (Figure 14.4). TF binds to activated factor VII, forming TF–VIIa complexes; the mechanism of activation of factor VII is unclear. The TF–VIIa complexes bind and activate factors IX to IXa and X to Xa. Factor IXa activates factor X. Factor Xa then attaches to the platelet surface and acts on prothrombin (factor II) to generate small

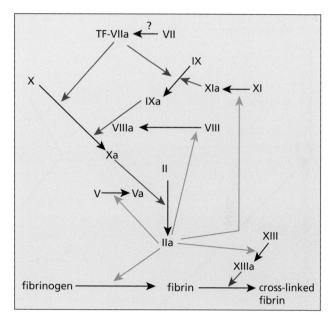

Figure 14.4 Pathways involved in fibrin generation after the activation of coagulation *in vivo* by TF. The suffix 'a' denotes the active form of each coagulation factor. *Notes*: Green arrows – actions of thrombin; red arrows – actions of other active enzymes; dashed blue arrows – inhibition.

amounts of thrombin (factor IIa). This pathway of thrombin generation is rapidly suppressed by tissue factor pathway inhibitor (TFPI). The small amount of thrombin generated activates the cofactors VIII, V and the zymogen factor XI as well as platelets. Factor XIa converts more factor IX to IXa. Factor VIIIa enhances the activity of factor IXa formed by the action of TF–VIIa complexes and factor XIa on factor IX, and markedly amplifies the conversion of factor X to Xa and, consequently, the generation of thrombin from prothrombin, which is augmented by factor Va. Thrombin splits two small negatively charged peptide fragments (fibrinopeptides A and B) from fibrinogen (factor I), thus removing repulsive forces from the molecule and allowing the remainder to polymerize and form the fibrin fibre. Finally, factor XIIIa, generated by the activation of factor XIII by thrombin, stabilizes and strengthens the fibrin polymers by forming covalent bonds between the fibrin chains (glutamine–lysine bridges). Calcium is required at several stages in the coagulation sequence. The reactions involving factors IXa, VIIIa and X to form Xa (tenase reaction) and factors Xa, Va and II to form IIa (prothrombinase reaction) take place mainly on the exposed phospholipids on the surface of platelets; the rate of reaction at the surface is considerably higher than that in solution. Hence bleeding in thrombocytopenia results from a failure of the clotting cascade as well as the lack of a platelet plug.

The extent of thrombin generation is limited by a number of natural anticoagulant mechanisms. Thrombin binds to thrombomodulin on the endothelial cell surface and the resulting complex activates protein C (PC) to activated protein C (APC), which inactivates factors Va and VIIIa in the presence of a cofactor protein S (Figure 14.8). In addition, free thrombin is directly inactivated by the circulating inhibitor antithrombin (AT), after the latter binds to heparans on endothelial cells.

Previous *in vitro* studies identified two pathways or systems within the coagulation cascade: a so-called intrinsic system, all the components of which are in the plasma, and a so-called extrinsic system consisting of TF, factor VII, factor X (with V as the cofactor), factor II and factor I. The sequence of action of factors in the intrinsic system was considered to be XII, XI, IX (with VIII as the cofactor), X (with V as the cofactor), II and I, as illustrated in Figure 14.5. The clotting sequence was initiated *in vitro* by activation of factor XII. Following limited activation, factor XII converts the plasma protein prekallikrein to kallikrein, which in turn activates factor XII fully to XIIa. Another plasma protein, high molecular weight kininogen, is a non-enzymatic accelerator of these interactions. Factor XIIa then acts on XI to form the active enzyme XIa. This is not the physiological pathway for the initiation of coagulation *in vivo* as shown by the absence of a bleeding tendency in people with an inherited deficiency of factor XII. However, the intrinsic/extrinsic system model remains valuable in understanding laboratory tests for blood coagulation (Figure 14.5).

Six of the synonyms for the factors are still in general use and should be known. They are antihaemophilic

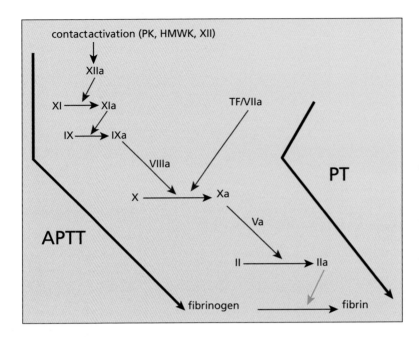

Figure 14.5 The sequence of coagulation *in vitro* brought about by by either contact activation of factor XII or by addition of tissue factor. The suffix 'a' denotes the active form of each coagulation factor. The former is the basis of the activated partial thromboplastin time (APTT) and the latter the prothrombin time (PT).

globulin (factor VIII), Christmas factor (factor IX), prothrombin and thrombin (factor II and IIa) and fibrinogen (now rarely referred to as factor I).

The fibrinolytic mechanism

After haemostasis has been achieved, the body has a mechanism for the enzymatic lysis of clots (Figure 14.6). The dissolution of the fibrin into fibrin-degradation products (FDPs) is carried out by the proteolytic plasma enzyme plasmin. Plasmin is present in the plasma in an inactive form, plasminogen, which is synthesized in the liver; plasminogen

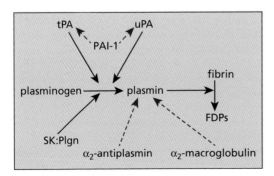

Figure 14.6 The fibrinolytic mechanism.

binds to fibrin and is converted to plasmin mainly by fibrin-bound tissue plasminogen activator (t-PA), which is synthesized and released by the injured vascular endothelium. Small amounts of plasmin are also generated from plasminogen by urokinase, which is produced mainly by renal cells but also other cell types such as endothelial cells. Bradykinin, which is released from high molecular weight kininogen by the action of kallikrein, is a powerful stimulator of t-PA release. The plasma contains an inhibitor of t-PA known as plasminogen activator inhibitor-1 (PAI-1).

Plasmin is not specific for fibrin, but can also break down other protein components of plasma, including fibrinogen and the clotting factors Va and VIIIa, and thus the following mechanism is present to confine the activities of plasmin to fibrin. When fibrin is formed, t-PA and plasminogen are specifically adsorbed onto fibrin; the t-PA–fibrin complex has a high affinity for plasminogen and converts it to plasmin, which digests the fibrin to which it is adsorbed. Under normal conditions, any plasmin released from the fibrin into the circulation is immediately inactivated by combining with the liver-derived plasma inhibitors, α_2-antiplasmin and α_2-macroglobulin. In this way, generalized breakdown of fibrinogen and other proteins does not occur.

Available thrombolytic drugs include urokinase and recombinant t-PAs as well as non-physiological activators, such as streptokinase, derived from certain streptococci and anisoylated plasminogen–streptokinase activator complex (APSAC). Recombinant t-PAs (alteplase, reteplase and tenecteplase) and streptokinase are the most frequently used drugs and are administered intravenously for the treatment of early acute myocardial infarction. Thrombolytic drugs may also be useful in other types of thrombosis.

Tests for clotting defects

There are three basic tests that are widely used, all performed on platelet-poor plasma obtained by centrifugation:

1 The *activated partial thromboplastin time* (APTT), which estimates the activity of factors XII, XI, IX, VIII, X, V, II and fibrinogen (the 'intrinsic system'; Figure 14.5).
2 The *prothrombin time* (PT), which estimates the activity of factors VII, X, V, II and fibrinogen (the 'extrinsic system'; Figure 14.5).
3 The *thrombin time*, adding thrombin to plasma and measuring the time taken to clot, which is prolonged when there is an inherited or acquired deficiency of fibrinogen, or an inherited or acquired abnormal fibrinogen molecule (dysfibrinogenaemia) or in the presence of heparin or raised levels of FDPs.

It is evident from Figure 14.5 that deficiencies of factors X, V, prothrombin (factor II) or fibrinogen will cause prolongations of both the APTT and PT. Patients with liver disease or DIC who have acquired deficiencies of several factors show prolongation of both the APTT and PT. Patients with acquired deficiencies of factors II, VII, IX and X (vitamin K-dependent factors), resulting from treatment with coumarin drugs or from vitamin K deficiency (p. 129), also have a prolonged APTT and PT. The PT is more sensitive than the APTT in detecting these deficiencies because of the short half-life of factor VII. In the small group of patients with congenital defects of one of the clotting factors, 80–90% have haemophilia (factor VIII deficiency), about 10–20% have factor IX deficiency, and only about 1% have deficiencies of one of the other eight factors. In haemophilia A and B the APTT is prolonged and the PT is normal. By determining both the APTT and the PT it is possible to obtain information as to where the defect lies.

Activated partial thromboplastin time

There is a wide range in the time taken for venous blood to clot in a glass tube at 37 °C. This wide range in the whole blood clotting time is due to two variables. First, activation of factor XII by the glass surface is variable and depends on such factors as the type of glass. Second, there is a variation in the coagulation-potentiating activities supplied by the platelets, as platelet numbers vary considerably between individuals. In the APPT addition of a phospholipid (partial thromboplastin) replaces the platelets and the variation in contact activation is substantially abolished by the addition of a contact activator (such as kaolin or micronized silica). The test is simple to carry out. Citrated plasma (which does not clot because of a lack of calcium) is obtained and to this is added a mixture of contact activator and phospholipid followed by calcium, and the time taken for the mixture to clot is measured. Prolongation of the clotting time is often due to a deficiency of factors VIII and IX (provided that a deficiency of factor X onwards has been excluded by a normal PT) and the test is sufficiently sensitive to detect deficiencies of both these factors when their concentration is reduced to 30% or less of the normal value; that is, it will detect the patients with mild haemophilia who only have severe bleeding after minor surgical procedures. An isolated prolonged APTT may also be due to factor XI deficiency, a contact factor (factor XII, pre-kallikrein, high molecular weight kininogen) deficiency, or a lupus anticoagulant (p. 131). Contact factor deficiency and lupus anticoagulants do not cause bleeding

Prothrombin time

The test used to measure the integrity of the extrinsic system is the one-stage PT. This test is carried out by adding tissue thromboplastin (TF and phospholipid) together with calcium to citrated plasma. Reference to Figure 14.5 shows that TF and factor VII (actually the TF–VIIa complex) initiate coagulation by activating factor X to Xa and hence prolongation of the PT results from deficiencies of I, II, V, VII and X. The PT is thus a misnomer, as deficiency of at least five factors affects the test and prothrombin deficiency alone must be gross before the PT is prolonged. The test is chiefly sensitive to deficiencies of factors V, VII and X.

When the PT is used for the control of oral anticoagulant therapy, the results are expressed as the international normalized ratio (INR). This is derived from the PT ratio (i.e. the patient's PT:mean normal PT) and a factor determined for each thromboplastin reagent by comparing its activity against an international reference preparation. The value of using the INR is that for patients taking vitamin K antagonists, the same therapeutic ranges apply irrespective of the source of thromboplastin.

Congenital coagulation disorders

Blood clotting abnormalities can be conveniently divided into two categories, congenital defects and acquired defects. This section deals with those that are present from birth.

There is a group of patients who complain of excessive bleeding, either spontaneous or following trauma, usually starting early in life, and who frequently have a family history of a similar condition. These patients usually have one of three diseases: haemophilia A, haemophilia B or VWD.

Haemophilia A (factor VIII deficiency)

The term 'haemophilia', first used by Schönlein in 1839, was applied to a lifelong tendency to prolonged haemorrhage found in males and dependent on the transmission of a sex-linked abnormal gene. During the decade 1950–60, it was found that there are in fact two diseases within the group of patients who, on clinical and genetic grounds, had been diagnosed as having haemophilia: patients with factor VIII deficiency and those with factor IX deficiency.

Genetics, prevalence and biochemistry

Deficiency of factor VIII results from an abnormality in the factor VIII gene, which is very large (186 kilobases, 26 exons) and lies at the tip of the long arm of the X-chromosome. Various abnormalities in the nucleotide sequence of this gene have been identified in about half the cases of haemophilia, ranging from single-point mutations to large deletions. Half of all severe cases are due to an inversion involving intron 22. The disease is almost entirely confined to hemizygous males, since the normal X-chromosome in heterozygous females is almost always capable of bringing about adequate factor VIII production. The prevalence of this disorder is about one per 10 000 males. Females with haemophilia have been observed extremely rarely and these are either homozygotes for the abnormal gene or are heterozygotes in whom the normal X-chromosome has not produced sufficient quantities of factor VIII due to lyonization. Daughters of males with haemophilia are obligatory carriers of the gene, since they must inherit the abnormal X-chromosome. Sons, on the other hand, are always normal, since they inherit the Y-chromosome. A female with a genetic defect on one X-chromosome will transmit the disease to half her sons, and half her daughters will become carriers. Patients suspected of having haemophilia should be carefully questioned for a history of a bleeding disorder occurring in the relations on the maternal side as opposed to the paternal side. There is a steady spontaneous mutation rate of the gene responsible for factor VIII production, since approximately one third of all people with haemophilia have no family history of the disease; this has been corroborated by studies on the genomic DNA.

The factor VIII molecule is a protein with a molecular weight of 8×10^4 daltons. In the plasma, factor VIII is only found complexed with VWF, which acts as a carrier and prolongs its plasma half-life. The factor VIII coagulant activity can be measured biologically by its ability to act as a cofactor to factor IXa (see Figure 14.4). Although factor VIII coagulant activity is greatly depressed in haemophilia, the amount of VWF is within normal limits.

Detection of carriers and antenatal diagnosis

Female carriers on average have half the clotting activity per unit of VWF compared to normal, however discrimination between cariers and non-carriers is often not possible based on factor assays alone. Genetic mutational analysis allows carriers to be identified with accuracy and is the method of choice.

Prenatal diagnosis of haemophilia can be made by analysis of fetal DNA, which can be obtained either by chorionic villus sampling between 11½ and 14 weeks of gestation or by amniocentesis after 16 weeks.

Clinical features

The characteristic clinical feature of severe haemophilia is the occurrence of spontaneous bleeding into the joints (Figure 14.7) and less frequently into the muscles; these two sites account for about 95% of all bleeds requiring treatment (Table 14.2). The presenting symptom is pain in the affected area and this can be very severe. Haemophiliacs rapidly become expert at diagnosing the onset of haemorrhage in its earliest stages, allowing treatment to be initiated at a time when it can be most effective. If not properly treated, bleeding into joints results in crippling deformity. The knees, elbows and ankles are most commonly affected. Haematuria, epistaxis and gastrointestinal bleeding are less common. Intracranial bleeding is the most common cause of death from the disease itself (i.e. discounting deaths from HIV infection — see below), accounting for

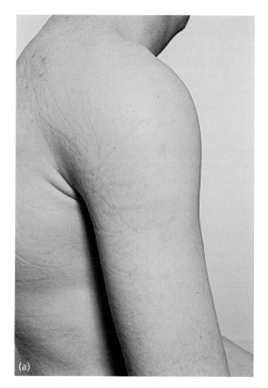
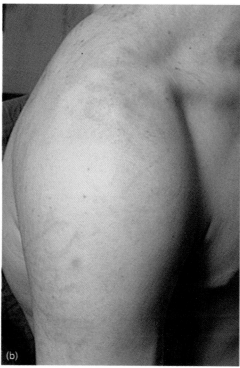

(a) (b)

Figure 14.7 Haemarthrosis of the shoulder joint in a patient with haemophilia A.

25–30% of all such deaths; only about one-half of the affected patients have a history of trauma.

The severity of bleeding and mode of presentation are related to the level of plasma factor VIII; this relationship is shown in Table 14.3. The severity of the disease often remains constant throughout a family.

Because of treatment with HIV-contaminated factor VIII concentrates between about 1978 and 1985, over 50% of patients with severe haemophilia in the USA and Europe became HIV positive; many of these have died of the acquired immune deficiency syndrome (AIDS). In addition, virtually all people treated for severe haemophilia before 1985 were infected with hepatitis C virus due to the use of non-virally inactivated factor concentrates.

Table 14.2 **The frequency of bleeding sites in 207 haemophiliacs.**

Lesion or operation	Percentage
Haemarthroses	79
Muscle haematomas	15
Haematuria Epistaxes Gastrointestinal bleeding Dental extraction Major surgery	Each about 1–2 Total 6

Source: From Rizza (1977) Br. Med. Bull. 33, 225–30.

Table 14.3 **The relation between plasma factor VIII levels and severity of bleeding.**

Factor VIII level (units/100 mL)	Bleeding symptoms
50	None
25–50	Excessive bleeding after major surgery or serious accident (often not diagnosed until incident occurs)
5–25	Excessive bleeding after minor surgery and injuries
1–5	Severe bleeding after minor surgery (sometimes spontaneous haemorrhage)
0	Spontaneous bleeding into muscles and joints

Source: From Rizza (1977) Br. Med. Bull. 33, 225–30.

Diagnosis

The possibility of haemophilia is suggested by the finding of a normal PT and a prolonged APTT. Confirmation is by a specific assay of factor VIII coagulant activity with normal VWF. The combination of a normal PT and a prolonged APTT is most often caused by lupus anticoagulant (see p. 131).

Treatment

Treatment should be given at the earliest sign of spontaneous or post-traumatic bleeding. It should also be given prophylactically if any type of operation is contemplated. Treatment consists of intravenous injections of virucidally treated plasma-derived high-purity factor VIII concentrate or recombinant factor VIII preparations to maintain plasma factor VIII coagulant activity to between 30% and 100% of normal, depending on the severity of the injury or extent of the proposed surgical procedure. In general, the more extensive the bleeding or degree of trauma, the larger the dose of factor VIII concentrate that is required. HIV has been eliminated from currently used plasma-derived factor VIII preparations by using donors who do not have HIV antibodies and by employing one or more virucidal methods (e.g. heating the lyophilized product at 80 °C, heating in solution at 60 °C or adding a solvent detergent mixture during the manufacturing process). Most developed countries have switched to recombinant products. Frequent assays of factor VIII levels in the plasma may be necessary to ensure that the concentration is being maintained at the appropriate level.

Approximately 25% of patients with haemophilia, usually after treatment with factor VIII on 10–20 occasions, develop antibodies that inhibit its functional activity and in 5-10% of patients these are of high titre. Haemorrhage in patients with high-titre inhibitors may require treatment with 'bypassing agents' such as recombinant factor VIIa or FEIBA (factor eight inhibitor bypassing activity; that is, a plasma-derived activated prothrombin complex concentrate), which activate the coagulation cascade below the level of factor VIII.

The administration of factor VIII may be avoided in mild to moderate haemophilia by using the vasopressin analogue desmopressin (DDAVP), which causes a temporary increase in factor VIII and VWF by provoking the release of these factors from endothelial cells. DDAVP is used intravenously, subcutaneously or intranasally. The antifibrinolytic drug tranexamic acid should be administered with DDAVP, as the latter also causes release of t-PA from the endothelium.

Freeze-dried factor VIII concentrates can be stored for prolonged periods and can be injected in adequate amounts in a small volume. This has made it possible for many patients to be treated at home by self-administration, thus allowing factor VIII to be injected as soon as symptoms appear. Such early therapy results in both rapid cessation of bleeding and rapid recovery. As an extension to this, many severely affected patients receive regular prophylactic treatment with factor VIII.

Haemophilia B (Factor IX deficiency, Christmas disease)

The differentiation of factor IX deficiency from factor VIII deficiency was first made by Biggs and colleagues in 1952. The clinical features and inheritance of factor IX deficiency are identical to those in factor VIII deficiency. Factor IX deficiency affects about 1 in every 50 000 males (i.e. it is less frequent than factor VIII deficiency). The factor IX gene is located on the long arm of the X-chromosome, is much smaller than the factor VIII gene (containing eight exons) and has been fully sequenced. Mutations in this gene have been found in virtually all cases of factor IX deficiency.

The APTT is prolonged and the PT normal. The diagnosis can be made by assay of the factor IX level. Plasma-derived factor IX concentrate or recombinant factor IX is available and should be administered intravenously as soon as spontaneous or post-traumatic bleeding starts. Factor IX has a longer half-life in the plasma (18–24 hours) than factor VIII and hence can be given at less frequent intervals.

Von Willebrand disease

This is the most common inherited bleeding disorder, with a prevalence of up to 1%, although most mild cases are undiagnosed. It was described by von Willebrand in 1926 as occurring in several families on islands in the Baltic (Åland Islands). It is an autosomal disoder characterized by mild, moderate or severe bleeding. The bleeding results from either a qualitative abnormality or a deficiency of VWF. This factor is a protein with a molecular weight of 2.7×10^5 daltons and exists in the plasma as a variable-sized polymer, ranging from a dimer to a molecule containing 50–100 subunits. It has a dual function: first, it is an adhesive molecule that binds platelets to subendothelial tissues; second, it acts as a carrier for factor VIII. The reduction in VWF results in a reduction in factor VIII concentration (usually measured as clotting activity), which may be as low as 5–30% of normal, similar to that found in mild haemophilia. The excessive bleeding in the disease is mainly due to the failure of the platelets to adhere rather than the concomitant factor VIII deficiency. An additional finding is that, whereas the antibiotic ristocetin induces platelet aggregation in platelet-rich plasma from normal subjects, it fails to do so in platelet-rich plasma from people with severe VWD. This observation is the basis of a useful laboratory test for the diagnosis of this disease.

The gene for VWF is present on chromosome 12 and analysis of the gene has shown that there is considerable heterogeneity in the genetic defects found in VWD. Some defects result in a reduction in the plasma concentration of structurally normal VWF molecules, but others cause different qualitative abnormalities in the VWF molecule. VWD has been divided into three types: in types 1 (most frequent) and 3 there is a partial reduction or nearly complete absence of VWF molecules, respectively, and in type 2 there are qualitative abnormalities.

Most patients have type 1 VWD, inherited as an autosomal dominant trait with variable penetrance, and are mildly affected. Spontaneous bleeding is usually confined to mucous membranes and skin and takes the form of epistaxes and ecchymoses, bleeding after dental extraction and menorrhagia. Severe haemorrhage may occur following surgical procedures. Bleeding into joints and muscles is rare except in type 3 disease.

The laboratory findings include a prolonged PFA closure time (if done), usually a prolonged APTT and reduced factor VIII clotting activity, reduced levels of VWF and impaired ristocetin-induced platelet aggregation; however, it is important to remember that the PFA and APTT may be within normal limits.

For mildly or moderately affected patients with type 1 disease, desmopressin (DDAVP), which increases plasma levels of both VWF and factor VIII, should be tried before using blood products. In unresponsive patients, intermediate purity factor VIII concentrates that contain VWF and factor VIII are effective in stopping haemorrhage, mainly by correcting the bleeding time but also by increasing factor VIII clotting activity, which continues to increase for many hours after treatment. Alternatively, very high-purity VWF concentrate may be used. High-purity factor VIII concentrates are unsuitable for the treatment of VWD since they contain very little VWF. The antifibrinolytic drug tranexamic acid may be used for treating epistaxis or menorrhagia and in combination with DDAVP or VWF-containing concentrates to manage dental extractions.

Deficiency of other clotting factors

Single deficiencies of factors other than VIII and IX are very rare, but all possible deficiencies have been found and all except contact factor (e.g. factor XII) deficiency give rise to bleeding disorders of varying degrees of severity. The explanation for the absence of excessive haemorrhage in factor XII deficiency is that the physiological activator of factor IX is thrombin, not factor XII (see Figure 14.4).

Acquired coagulation disorders

The hepatocytes are the major cell type involved in the synthesis of all the coagulation factors. Hence, severe liver disease may result in bleeding, due both to a deficiency of several coagulation factors and to an abnormality in the structure and function of fibrinogen, as well as thrombocytopenia due to hypersplenism.

The final stages in the synthesis of factors II, VII, IX and X (collectively known as the prothrombin group or complex) involve a vitamin K-dependent carboxylase, which adds carboxyl (–COOH) groups to the proteins; these groups are necessary for the efficient functioning of the molecules.

The coumarin drugs are vitamin K antagonists and their administration results in only partial carboxylation of the prothrombin group of coagulation factors, which are consequently considerably less active than normal in the clotting cascade. Similar abnormalities are seen in vitamin K deficiency, which may be found in the newborn (haemorrhagic disease of the newborn), in patients with intestinal malabsorption and, since bile salts are required for vitamin K absorption, also in patients with biliary obstruction or biliary fistulae. Examination of Figure 14.5 shows that except for factor IX, the clotting factors involved in these acquired deficiencies are detected by the PT and that apart from factor VII, they are also detected by the APTT. However, as mentioned earlier, the PT is the more sensitive test due to the short half-life of factor VII and, consequently, it is the test employed for monitoring oral anticoagulant therapy and detecting the abnormalities in vitamin K deficiency.

Disseminated intravascular coagulation (DIC)

DIC describes a process in which there is a generalized activation of the clotting system followed by marked activation of the fibrinolytic system. Acute DIC may be associated with premature separation of the placenta (abruptio placentae), amniotic fluid embolism or shock, and may also be seen in certain bacterial infections such as meningococcal septicaemia, where the endotoxin causes damage to monocytes and vascular endothelium. It is a common complication following intravascular haemolysis of red cells after a mismatched transfusion. The syndrome also occurs occasionally after extensive accidental or surgical trauma, particularly following thoracic operations. Chronic DIC is seen when there is retention of a dead fetus as well as in patients with disseminated carcinoma, lymphoma and leukaemia (especially acute promyelocytic leukaemia). Other clinical associations of DIC include purpura fulminans (following scarlet fever, chickenpox or rubella), brain injuries, extensive burns, liver disease and snake bites.

In those diseases that are associated with DIC, the clotting cascade may be activated in various ways; namely, by the release of TF from damaged tissues, monocytes or red cells; by damage to endothelial cells; and by abnormal activators of coagulation. Activation of the cascade leads to the generation and dissemination of large amounts of thrombin in the circulation, the activation of platelets and the formation of intravascular microthrombi. If this is sufficiently extensive, there is a reduction of the concentration of fibrinogen and other clotting factors in the plasma, which impairs haemostatic activity. As a consequence of the fibrin formation, the fibrinolytic mechanism is activated (p. 122), resulting in high concentrations of FDPs, including D-dimers. This leads to further haemostatic impairment, since FDPs inhibit fibrin clot formation by interfering with the polymerization of the fibrin monomer. FDPs also interfere with the aggregation of platelets. With continued intravascular coagulation, there is increased expression of thrombomodulin on endothelial cells and the thrombin–thrombomodulin complexes activate protein C; APC inactivates factors Va and VIIIa, further aggravating the haemostatic defect, and also inhibits PAI-1, which stimulates fibrinolysis. The end result is generalized haemorrhage due to failure of haemostasis.

The haemorrhagic manifestations may be so severe in acute DIC as to lead to death. They include petechiae, ecchymoses and bleeding from the nose, mouth, urinary and gastrointestinal tracts and vagina. Haemorrhage may also occur into the pituitary gland, liver, adrenals and brain. Although the usual clinical manifestation of acute DIC is haemorrhage, occasionally the clinical picture is dominated by signs and symptoms of widespread thrombosis and infarction; thrombi are most frequently found in the microvasculature. There may be digital gangrene, adult respiratory distress syndrome, neurological signs and renal failure. Mild hypotension is commonly present in acute DIC and may progress to become more severe and irreversible if not treated in time.

In chronic DIC, the haemorrhagic tendency may be mild or moderate. However, some patients with chronic DIC are asymptomatic because the activation of the clotting and fibrinolytic systems is finely balanced and the production of clotting factors and platelets is sufficiently increased to compensate for their increased consumption.

Diagnosis

This is partly dependent on being aware of the conditions with which DIC is associated. The investigations of value in the diagnosis of acute or chronic DIC are as follows:

- *The platelet count*: Platelets become enmeshed in the fibrin clots on the vascular endothelium and thrombocytopenia is an early and common sign.
- *The APTT and the PT*: These are usually prolonged, due to the depletion of clotting factors, especially in acute DIC.
- *The fibrinogen concentration*: This is reduced. The best method for the estimation of fibrinogen is based on the time taken for a diluted sample of plasma to clot in the presence of high concentrations of thrombin (the Clauss method).
- *The thrombin time*: This may be prolonged due to a combination of a low fibrinogen and excessive amounts of FDPs (which inhibit fibrin polymerization). The thrombin time is determined by adding low concentrations of thrombin to citrated plasma and measuring the time for the appearance of a clot.
- *Estimation of FDPs using the D-dimer assay*: FDPs including D-dimers are increased. D-dimers can be detected by rapid immunological tests in which latex particles coated with monoclonal antibody directed against D-dimer are agglutinated by D-dimers present in plasma.

Treatment

Since the activation of the clotting system is the primary initiating stimulus and fibrinolysis is mainly a secondary phenomenon, treatment is aimed at preventing further coagulation by removal of the initiating cause (e.g. when it occurs in obstetric practice, rapid and non-traumatic vaginal delivery stops the clotting process). While the initiating cause is being dealt with, patients with acute DIC should be supported with transfusions of blood, fresh-frozen plasma and plate-let concentrates in order to restore blood volume and replace clotting factors and platelets.

Acquired haemophilia

A rare but devastating acquired bleeding disorder is due to autoantibody-mediated factor VIII deficiency. It can occur in either sex, is more common in the elderly and has a high mortality. It is treated with 'by-passing agents' such as recombinant factor VIIa or FEIBA (see above) and immune suppression.

Anticoagulant drugs

The two most frequently used anticoagulant drugs are heparin and vitamin K antagonists such as warfarin. Parenteral heparin is used in patients with deep vein thrombosis (DVT) or pulmonary embolism (PE) and is followed by oral warfarin therapy. Subcutaneous heparin is used to reduce the risk of DVT and PE in hospitalized patients, including those undergoing surgery (especially hip surgery). Heparin does not cross the placenta and is therefore the preferred drug when anticoagulation is required during pregnancy. The oral anticoagulant warfarin is administered ini-tially for three months to patients with DVT or PE and may be indicated long term to prevent recurrent venous thrombosis. Long-term warfarin is also used after the insertion of mechanical heart valves and in patients with atrial fibrillation.

Heparin

Standard unfractionated heparin is an acidic muco-polysaccharide (average molecular weight 1.5×10^4 daltons) that has to be administered intravenously or subcutaneously. When administered intravenously, its biological half-life is 1 h. Heparin potentiates the action of AT, a molecule that inactivates the activated serine protease coagulation factors thrombin (IIa) and Xa. Heparin chains longer than 18 saccharides in length can link AT and IIa molecules leading to pow-erful inhibition; shorter chains act predominantly by potentiating the action against Xa. Low molecular weight heparin (average molecular weight $4–5 \times 10^3$ daltons) is used subcutaneously, it inactivates Xa to a greater extent than IIa and has a longer biological half-life. Examples of low molecular weight heparins currently in use are dalteparin, enoxaparin and tin-zaparin. Fondaparinux is a synthetic pentasaccharide that induces AT specifically to inhibit Xa.

For the treatment of thrombosis or embolism, standard heparin may be administered as a bolus of 5000 units (70 units/kg) intravenously, followed by a continuous intravenous infusion of 15–25 units/kg/h. Treatment is monitored by performing the APTT, the heparin dosage being altered so as to maintain the APTT at 1.5–2.5 times the normal value, although these figures may vary with different APTT reagents. However, the treatment of choice is now low molecu-lar weight heparin given subcutaneously once a day with no monitoring (because of the high predictabil-ity of effect when given according to body weight). When a patient with venous thromboembolism un-dergoing treatment with heparin is started on war-farin, the heparin should be given for at least 5 days or until the INR has been therapeutic for at least 24 hours, whichever is the longer.

Either standard or, more usually, low molecu-lar weight heparin is administered subcutaneously to prevent venous thrombosis in hospitalized pa-tients at risk of thrombosis. The dosage of standard heparin for prevention of postoperative thrombosis is 5000 units subcutaneously preoperatively, followed by 5000 units subcutaneously 8–12 hourly; low mo-lecular weight heparin is administered once daily.

Haemorrhage due to overdosage is managed by stopping the heparin and, if necessary, by giving protamine sulphate intravenously. Side effects of heparin include heparin-induced thrombocytopenia (HIT) via an antibody-based mechanism (see p. 119), osteoporosis (following long-term use), alopecia and hypersensitivity reactions.

Warfarin sodium

This is a coumarin derivative that is administered orally once a day. As has already been mentioned, it is a vitamin K antagonist and interferes with the car-boxylation and hence with the functional activity of factors II, VII, IX and X, protein C and protein S. After the first dose, clotting factor activity is reduced in the order VII, IX, X and II (i.e. the factor with the shortest half-life is reduced fastest and the longest half-life most slowly).

It is customary to prescribe 5 or 10 mg warfarin on the first day and subsequent doses are based on the INR. The therapeutic range for the INR is usually 2–3. A higher range of 3–4 is used for recurrent DVT or PE, despite an INR >2 and for patients with certain prosthetic heart valves.

There are many possible causes for loss of control of warfarin therapy, including the simultaneous use of drugs that affect warfarin metabolism by cytochrome P450 and changes in dietary vitamin K. Bleeding is controlled by stopping the warfarin by administering vitamin K and, if necessary, administering prothrombin complex concentrates.

Warfarin crosses the placenta and may cause developmental abnormalities such as chondrodysplasia, microcephaly and blindness. It is therefore contraindicated in the first trimester of pregnancy. It should also not be administered during the last few weeks of pregnancy because of its anticoagulant effect on the fetus and the consequent risk of fetal or placental haemorrhage.

Direct oral thrombin inhibitors and direct oral Xa inhibitors

Drugs that directly inhibit thrombin (e.g. dabiagtran etexilate) or Xa (e.g. rivaroxaban, apixaban, edoxaban) have been developed as oral anticoagulants that offer an alternative to warfarin in the treatment of venous thromboembolism and atrial fibrillation. They can be given in fixed dose without monitoring; they have relatively short half-lives (in the order of 9–17 hours) but no antidote.

Investigation of a patient with abnormal bleeding

A most important step in the diagnostic process is taking a good history from the patient. The physician should ask, among others, the following questions: Has the patient ever bled excessively in the past and have any relatives bled excessively? More specifically, has the patient had tonsillectomy, major abdominal or orthopaedic surgery or dental extractions in the past, and if so, was there any abnormal bleeding? The relationship between the type of bleeding and the nature of the haemostatic defect has been discussed earlier (p. 115).

The screening tests that are useful in investigating a patient who gives a history of excessive bleeding are the following:

- A blood count, including a platelet count, and examination of a blood film.
- The prothrombin time and the activated partial thromboplastin time.
- The thrombin time or fibrinogen assay.

The PFA 100 can be used as a screening test for abnormal platelet function, but if diagnostic suspicion is high, platelet aggregation studies must be performed. If any of these tests is found to be abnormal, further

specialized tests may be necessary. The screening tests do not reliably exclude VWD and, if suspected, specific tests should be done.

Natural anticoagulant mechanisms and the prothrombotic state (thrombophilia)

There are natural anticoagulant mechanisms in the plasma that prevent localized fibrin formation from becoming widespread. The most important molecules involved in these mechanisms are AT, protein C and protein S, all of which are produced in the liver. Inherited or acquired abnormalities of these inhibitors of coagulation may lead to a prothrombotic state (thrombophilia). This section summarizes the essential information relating to (i) the congenital deficiency of these factors; (ii) prothrombotic states due to the presence of a specific polymorphism in factor V (factor V Leiden) or prothrombin (G20210A polymorphism); and (iii) one acquired prothrombotic state known as the antiphospholipid syndrome.

Antithrombin

This is mainly an inhibitor of thrombin and factor Xa (Figure 14.8), but it also inhibits factors IXa and XIa and the TF–VIIa complex; its action is markedly potentiated by heparin. Normally some AT becomes activated by binding to endothelial cell-associated heparin sulphate and thus prevents thrombus formation on the endothelium. Congenital AT deficiency is inherited as an autosomal dominant char-

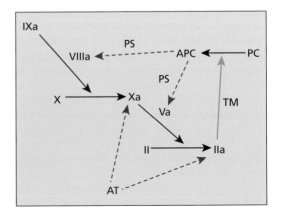

Figure 14.8 The natural anticoagulants.

acter; its prevalence is about 1 in 3000. There are a number of molecular variants of AT, with different degrees of risk of thrombosis. Heterozygotes (whose AT concentrations are 40–50% of normal) may suffer from recurrent DVT, mesenteric vein thrombosis and PE; the first thrombotic event usually occurs between the ages of 15 and 50 years. Homozygotes are rarely seen, presumably due to fetal wastage.

Protein C and protein S

Two other inhibitors of coagulation are the vitamin K-dependent substances protein C and protein S. Protein C becomes activated when it reacts with thrombin bound to thrombomodulin, a protein of the endothelial cell membrane. Activated protein C (APC) is a serine protease and degrades factors Va and VIIIa, in a reaction potentiated by its cofactor, protein S (Figure 14.8).

Some individuals have a hereditary deficiency of protein C, with about 50% of normal levels; these are heterozygotes for a mutation affecting the protein C gene and in one study were found with a prevalence of about 1 per 300. A proportion of such heterozygotes displays the clinical picture seen in inherited AT deficiency, but in addition are particularly prone to develop superficial thrombophlebitis, cerebral vein thrombosis and coumarin-induced skin necrosis. Homozygotes for the mutant gene are rare, and those who have virtually no protein C present with purpura fulminans or extensive thrombosis of visceral veins in the neonatal period.

The incidence of protein C deficiency in children and adults below the age of 45 years with recurrent venous thrombosis is about 5% and the incidence of protein S deficiency in this group is similar.

Factor V Leiden and APC resistance

A polymorphism in factor V at the APC cleavage site ($Arg^{506} \rightarrow Gln$) results in a FVa molecule resistance to degradation by APC. In white Caucasian populations, about 5% are heterozygous for this polymorphism, which is known as factor V Leiden (after its place of discovery). It is found in about 20% of cases of venous thrombosis. Heterozygotes have a five- to sevenfold increase in the risk of thrombosis and homozygotes a ten- to fiftyfold increase.

Prothrombin allele G20210A

Between 1% and 2% of the population have a G20210A polymorphism in the 3′untranslated region of the prothrombin gene that increases prothrombin levels. This increases the risk for venous thrombosis two- to fourfold.

The antiphospholipid syndrome

The antiphospholipid antibody syndrome is defined by the presence of antiphospholipid antibodies (either anticardiolipin antibodies, antibeta-2 glycoprotein I antibodies or lupus anticoagulant) associated with thrombosis or certain problems in pregnancy. Lupus anticoagulant prolongs the results of coagulation tests that depend on phospholipid (e.g. the APTT). Although these antibodies have an anticoagulant effect *in vitro*, they are associated with thromboses *in vivo*. Features of the antiphospholipid syndrome may include recurrent venous thromboses (most commonly DVT of the lower limbs), recurrent arterial thrombosis (most commonly stroke) and recurrent miscarriage (due to placental thrombosis and infarction). Thrombocytopenia is common. Antiphospholipid antibodies are found in some patients with SLE or other autoimmune disorders as well as in individuals with no other evidence of an immunological abnormality. Recent work on the mechanisms underlying the thrombotic tendency suggests that the relevant antibodies are those directed against $\beta 2$ glycoprotein I, these antibodies also being detected in the anticardiolipin ELISA ($\beta 2$ glycoprotein I, binds to negatively charged phospholipids) and in the lupus anticoagulant assay.

15

Blood groups and blood transfusion

Learning objectives

✓ To understand the inheritance and significance of the ABO system

✓ To understand the nature and significance of the Rh blood group system including RhD

✓ To know the principles involved in the selection of donor blood of suitable ABO and Rh groups for a recipient, and the principles of the cross-match, including the antiglobulin test

✓ To understand the hazards of blood transfusion (incompatible blood, allergic reactions, bacterial infection, citrate toxicity and transmission of disease) and of massive blood transfusion

✓ To know how to investigate a patient suspected of receiving an incompatible transfusion

✓ To know the basis of blood fractionation and the rationale for the use of specific blood products, including red cells, platelet concentrates, fresh-frozen plasma (FFP) and cryoprecipitate

✓ To know the pathogenesis, clinical features and the principles underlying the treatment and prevention of haemolytic disease of the newborn (HDN) due to anti-D

✓ To know the principles of antenatal care concerned with predicting both the presence and severity of HDN due to anti-D

✓ To know the differences between HDN due to anti-D and that due to anti-A and anti-B

Blood groups

One of the main problems in the transfusion of blood is the avoidance of immunological reactions resulting from the differences between donor and recipient red cells. Blood groups have arisen because mutations have occurred in the genes controlling the surface constituents of the red cells. These alterations in the surface structures have not usually affected the function of the red cell, but when the red cells of a donor are transfused into a recipient who lacks these antigens, they may induce an immunological response. There are 30 major blood group systems (e.g. the ABO group, Rh group), together giving hundreds of possible red cell phenotypes. Although all the systems

Haematology Lecture Notes, Ninth edition. C.S.R. Hatton, N.C. Hughes-Jones, D. Hay and D. Keeling. © 2013 John Wiley & Sons, Ltd.
Published 2013 by John Wiley & Sons, Ltd.

have given rise to transfusion difficulties (and in fact this is how they have been recognized), this chapter focuses on the two of greatest importance, the ABO and Rh systems.

ABO system

Practically all red cells have the H antigen, a carbohydrate group attached mainly to proteins on the cell membrane. This antigen is the basis for the ABO blood groups. The ABO locus is encoded on chromosome 9q, where one of three possible alleles may be found. The A allele encodes for a glycosyltransferase, which modifies the H antigen by adding N-acetylgalactosamine to it (thus forming the A antigen). The B allele of the ABO locus encodes an alternative glycosyltransferase that links galactose to the H antigen (thus converting it to the B antigen). The O allele, by contrast, encodes no functional enzyme at all, such that the H antigen remains unmodified. Since each patient inherits an allele of the ABO locus on each chromosome 9, there are six possible genotypes, namely AA, AO, BB, BO, AB and OO, and four possible phenotypes: A, AB, B and O. The frequency of these ABO group phenotypes differs in different populations; in the UK it is approximately group O, 46%; A, 42%; B, 9%; and AB, 3%.

Patients with group O blood (genotype O/O) will have only unmodified H antigen on their red cells, but will have circulating IgM antibodies to the A and B antigens. These antibodies exist even if the patient has never been exposed to blood of another group; they are thought to arise due to cross-reactivity between the ABO antigens and commonly seen epitopes in bacteria and/or food products, since they are produced universally in the first year of life. Transfusion of blood of group A or B to patients who have group O blood would therefore result in intravascular haemolysis of the transfused cells. Transfusion of group B blood to a patient of group A would have a similar effect; but group O blood, featuring only the universal H- antigen, should not produce a haemolytic response in patients of any ABO group. As such, it has been termed the 'universal donor' group. While the 'universal donor' label is true to some extent, it is also subject to caveats: group O blood may not contain an ABO antigen that will cause haemolysis, but in rare group O donors there may be the presence of high-titre antibodies against groups A and B, which themselves might induce passive haemolysis of the recipient's own red cells. This must be borne in mind when determining safe donor blood groups for specific recipients (see Table 15.1).

Table 15.1 Appropriate blood groups for transfusion.

Recipient blood group	Donor red cells	Donor plasma
A	A or O	A or AB
AB	A, B or O	AB only
B	B or O	B or AB
O	O only	A, B or O

Note: This table does not take account of other blood group antigens, and assumes that high-titre/atypical antibodies have been excluded from the donor unit.

It is the naturally occurring presence of anti-A and/or anti-B antibodies that makes ABO typing so critical to blood transfusion practice. Haemolytic reactions will occur immediately in the event of incompatible transfusion, and may be fatal (see complications of transfusion, below).

Rh system

The Rh system is also of great importance in transfusion medicine. It is frequently responsible for immunizing patients without the relevant antigen, and can cause problems with both transfusion and pregnancy.

The inheritance of the Rh blood group system is slightly more complex than that of the ABO system. Two separate genetic loci on chromosome 1 encode for a total of five antigens. The first locus, *RHD*, has alleles D or d; D encodes a transmembrane protein featuring the D antigen, while the allele d encodes a variant that does not bear this antigen. *RHCE* is an adjacent locus that encodes a transmembrane ion channel bearing the antigens C (or its variant, c) and E (or its variant, e). Alleles at this locus may be described as CE, Ce, cE and ce, denoting the set of antigens they encode. A complete description of the Rh haplotype for a patient will include alleles at both *RHD* and *RHCE* loci – for example, if a patient's full Rh genotype is DCe/DCE, they will have the RhD allele on both copies of chromosome 1, but Ce and CE alleles at the adjacent RHCE locus. They will therefore have the antigens D, C, E and e on their red cells. The commonest haplotypes are DCe, dce and DcE. The proximity of the two loci to each other means that meiotic crossing over is not seen, and the two loci are always inherited as a unit.

The D antigen is the most clinically important of the Rh group antigens, due to its high immunogenicity.

An RhD-negative person (e.g. dce/dce) has over a 50% chance of developing anti-D antibodies after the transfusion of one unit of RhD-positive blood: it is therefore important that RhD-negative patients receive RhD-negative blood. Exposure to the 'c' antigen will provoke anti-c production in only 2% of people lacking this antigen, such that the risk of immunization after giving blood of type dce/dce to an individual who lacks the 'c' antigen (for instance genotype DCe/DCe) is very small.

Note that unlike the ABO system, Rh antibodies are not naturally occurring; they must be raised by exposure of an antigen-negative individual to the appropriate antigen, either through transfusion of incompatible blood or through pregnancy. After the exposure, IgG antibodies come to predominate, and haemolysis is generally extravascular.

Other blood group systems

Other blood group antibodies, which are sometimes a problem during blood transfusion, include the following: anti-K (Kell system), anti-Fy^a (Duffy system), anti-Jk^a (Kidd system) and anti-S (part of the MNSs blood group system). These antigens are relatively poorly immunogenic. Their potency in stimulating antibody production is 10–1000 times less than that of RhD. Consequently, these antigens need not be routinely assessed prior to transfusion, although more care is required in patients who are on a chronic transfusion programme (e.g. in thalassaemia major), as the lifetime likelihood of immunization by these antigens is higher in heavily transfused patients.

Compatibility

The purpose of cross-matching blood before transfusion is to ensure that there is no antibody present in the recipient's plasma that will react with any antigen on the donor's cells. The basic technique for detecting such antibodies relies on their ability to agglutinate red cells that bear the appropriate antigen.

Unfortunately, many red cell antibodies are unable to bring about agglutination on their own; many require additional proteolytic treatment of the red cells or the use of an antiglobulin reagent (see below). The ability of antibodies to agglutinate untreated red cells depends partly on the molecular structure of the antibody. Pentameric IgM antibodies, which readily span adjacent red cells, can bring about agglutination without the addition of any other reagents. By contrast, the smaller IgG antibodies, which are far more common than IgM, do not usually cause agglutination.

Antiglobulin test

The antiglobulin test was first discovered by C. Moreschi in 1908, and its relevance to clinical practice was highlighted by R.R.A. Coombs, A.E. Mourant and R.R. Race in 1945. Its purpose is to detect antibodies to red cell surface constituents, either bound to the red cell surface or free in the serum.

The basic constituent of an antiglobulin serum is anti-human IgG, which is obtained by injecting human IgG into animals. Being bivalent, the antiglobulin is able to bring about agglutination of IgG-coated red cells by linking IgG molecules on one red cell with those on an adjacent red cell, thus holding the cells together as agglutinates.

The antiglobulin test can be used in two ways. First, it can be used to detect antibody already on the patient's cells *in vivo*. Red cells are washed to remove the free IgG in the plasma, which would otherwise react with and neutralize the antiglobulin. After washing, anti-human globin is added and, if the red cells are coated with antibody, agglutination takes place. This is the *direct antiglobulin test*, used in the diagnosis of autoimmune haemolytic anaemia and described in Chapter 3. Alternatively, the test can be used to detect the presence of antibody in serum, as in the cross-matching of blood for transfusion. In this case, serum from the patient who requires transfusion is incubated with donor red cells. Any antibody present in the recipient's serum that has specificity for antigens on the donor's cells will interact with those cells. After washing, addition of anti-human globulin will bring about red cell agglutination. This is *the indirect antiglobulin test*.

Procedure for obtaining compatible blood

The ABO and RhD group of the recipient must first be determined by the addition of agglutinating anti-A and anti-B to the red cells. The result is checked by determining whether anti-A or anti-B is present in the recipient's serum; this is done by adding known group A and B cells. Group A blood always contains anti-B in the plasma, group B blood has anti-A, and group O has anti-A and anti-B. The RhD group is also determined using an agglutinating IgM anti-D or by using IgG anti-D combined with the antiglobulin test.

Donor blood of the appropriate ABO and RhD group is then selected. Before this can be transfused, cross-matching must be carried out, partly to ensure that there have been no errors in the determination of the ABO group of the donor and recipient, and partly to ensure that no other antibodies are present in the recipient that react with the donor's red cells. A search is made for both agglutinating and non-agglutinating antibodies, the latter with the antiglobulin test.

The sera of all recipients will also be screened for the presence of antibodies such as anti-K (Kell), anti-Fyᵃ (Duffy) and anti-Jkᵃ (Kidd), using a panel of red cells of known phenotype. If screening is not carried out, these antibodies will be discovered in the final stages of a cross-matching procedure, using the antiglobulin test.

If RhD-negative donor blood is not available for RhD-negative recipients, the question arises whether it is safe to give RhD-positive blood. RhD-negative males, especially elderly males, may receive RhD-positive blood provided that care is taken to search for anti-RhD antibodies before any subsequent transfusions of RhD-positive blood are given. RhD-positive blood must never be given to RhD-negative girls or RhD-negative women of child-bearing potential, to avoid stimulating anti-D production with the risk of haemolytic disease of the newborn in subsequent pregnancies.

Haemolytic disease of the newborn

Haemolytic disease of the newborn (HDN) is a major example of the clinical significance of blood groups, and arises as a consequence of fetus and mother having different blood group antigens. Following the passage of fetal red cells across the placenta, there is immunization of the mother to fetal blood group antigens that she does not possess. The IgG antibodies produced are subsequently transferred back across the placenta, and react with the fetal red cells causing their destruction. Before the advent of prophylactic therapy, the overwhelming majority of cases were due to antibodies against the Rh-D antigen, with only 6% due to other antibodies within the Rh system and 1% due to antibodies in other blood group systems. Without treatment, the mortality rate of affected infants is about 20%, but antenatal prophylaxis together with the introduction of treatment by exchange transfusion, has considerably reduced this value. Approximately 60% of affected infants require an exchange transfusion and efficient treatment results in the survival of about 95% of all affected infants. During the decade 1958–68, the disease resulted in about 300–400 neonatal deaths each year in the United Kingdom, and an approximately equal number were stillborn. During the 1960s prophylactic anti-D immunoglobulin injections were routinely introduced

for RhD-negative mothers in the hours immediately following labour, to prevent active immunization due to fetal RhD exposure. Since then, the incidence of haemolytic disease of the newborn has been greatly reduced, and by the year 2000 only about 10–20 deaths occurred annually in the United Kingdom due to anti Rh-D HDN.

Haemolytic disease due to anti-D

The aetiology of HDN was first elucidated by Levine and colleagues in 1941. A mother who had given birth to an affected infant was transfused with her husband's blood and suffered a transfusion reaction. It was correctly surmised that the mother had been immunized by a fetal antigen that had been derived from the father. The Rh blood group system was also discovered during this period, and it was soon ascertained that the maternal antibody in this mother was anti-Rh, now known as anti-RhD.

Small numbers of fetal cells can occasionally be found in the maternal circulation throughout pregnancy, especially during the third trimester, but the main transplacental passage occurs at the time of labour. The volume of the haemorrhage is usually less than 5 mL, but occasionally may exceed 50 mL; there is evidence that the greater the number of fetal cells in the circulation, the greater the chance of developing antibodies. The relationship between the total amount of fetal red cells in the maternal circulation immediately after labour and the incidence of immunization of mothers six months later is shown in Table 15.2.

Table 15.2 The relationship between the number of fetal red cells in the maternal circulation after labour and the subsequent immunization of the mother.

Estimated number of fetal red cells (mL)	Incidence of immunization (%)
0	3.7
0.02	4.5
0.04	10.3
0.06–0.08	14.6
0.1–0.2	18.7
0.22–0.78	21.1
.0.8	23.5

Source: From Clarke (1968) Lancet ii, 1–7.

In the UK population, about 17% of women are RhD negative but, before the advent of preventive therapy, only about 6% of all D-negative women became immunized to the D antigen. This may be explained by the observation that not all fathers carry the D antigen; a substantial number of those who do are heterozygous, hence having only a 50% chance of transmitting the D allele. Furthermore, the amount of fetal red cells crossing the placenta is often insufficient to initiate immunization, and only about 60–70% of Rh-negative mothers are able to respond to the D-antigen by producing significant amounts of anti-D.

It is very unusual for the first-born child to be affected with HDN, the incidence being slightly less than 1% of all Rh-negative mothers who have no history of transfusion or abortion. The reason for this is that it is only occasionally that significant numbers of fetal red cells cross the placenta sufficiently early in pregnancy to stimulate anti-D production before the child is born.

If the fetal red cells in the mother after labour bring about a primary immunization, antibody may be found within the following six months. In about half of cases, however, antibody concentrations do not rise sufficiently high for anti-D to be detected at this time. During a subsequent pregnancy with an Rh-positive fetus, it only requires a few fetal red cells crossing the placenta early in pregnancy in order to provide a secondary stimulus to anti-D production. This can usually be detected by the 28th week but sometimes may not appear until the last few weeks of pregnancy.

Clinical features

There is a very great variation in the severity of the disease in an affected child. At one end of the scale there are infants who are not anaemic at birth and who never become jaundiced. However, the Hb concentration of these infants may fall abnormally rapidly after birth and values as low as 6 g/dL may be found up to 30 days later. All neonates with maternal antibodies on their red cells (positive direct antiglobulin test) should therefore be followed up for a short period after birth.

Moderately severely affected babies may or may not be anaemic at birth, but the rate of red cell destruction is such that jaundice develops within a few hours. Jaundice is not seen at the time of birth, since prior to this bilirubin is excreted by placental transfer. Within 48–72 hours of birth, the plasma bilirubin may rise to 350–700 μmol/L. The rate of rise of plasma bilirubin is governed partly by the rate of red cell destruction and partly by the degree of maturity of the bilirubin excretory mechanism. As a result of the poor development of the excretory mechanism for bilirubin in many infants, it is quite common for a child with a cord Hb within the normal range (lower limit 13.5 g/dL) to become severely jaundiced. The danger associated with a high bilirubin level is kernicterus resulting from damage to the basal ganglia of the brain, with a clinical picture characterized by spasticity and death from respiratory failure.

In the past, severely affected babies could become so anaemic that cardiac failure with hydrops, or even stillbirth would ensue. With modern management, such a severe clinical picture is rarely seen.

Management of mother and child

When a pregnant woman attends her first booking appointment with the antenatal service, she should have blood taken to check her ABO and RhD status, as well as to examine for any other red cell antibodies that might react with paternally derived antigens. Women who are negative for RhD are given routine antenatal anti-D prophylaxis at 28 weeks, 34 weeks and within 72 hours of delivery. This involves an intramuscular injection of anti-D immunoglobulin, which prevents active immunization in the case of red cell transfer across the placenta. In addition, any potentially sensitizing event is also treated with additional anti-D administration: such events include abdominal trauma, threatened abortion, or any spontaneous abortion after 12 weeks. An estimate of the size of any feto-maternal haemorrhage is permitted using the Kleihauer-Betke technique. This test exploits the differential sensitivity to acid of cells containing fetal haemoglobin and those containing adult globins. Treatment of a blood smear, taken from the mother's blood, with an acid preparation will leach only adult globin from the cells. The cells derived from the fetal circulation can then be counted, and the size of the feto-maternal haemorrhage defined. Appropriate titration of the correct dose of anti-D immunoglobulin can then be performed.

In pregnancies that are likely to be affected, ultrasound examination is useful to detect fetal hydrops and Doppler ultrasound of the middle cerebral artery can be used to assess fetal anaemia. If anaemia is confirmed by ultrasound-guided fetal blood sampling, intrauterine transfusion may be commenced. Since about half the total numbers of stillbirths occur after the 36th week of pregnancy, induction at 36 weeks reduces the incidence of stillbirth.

When anti-D is present in the mother's plasma, cord blood is obtained at delivery and the presence of antibody on the infant's red cells is confirmed by the direct antiglobulin test. Additional essential investigations include a full blood count and examination of the blood film for evidence of haemolysis, plus assessment of bilirubin levels.

The usual treatment of HDN involves exchange transfusion for neonates with severe anaemia and/or severe hyperbilirubinaemia (>350micromol/l) or rapidly increasing hyperbilirubinaemia. For less severe hyperbilirubinaemia, phototherapy can be effective in reducing the bilirubin by inducing photoisomerization to forms more readily excreted without the need for conjugation.

Haemolytic disease due to anti-A and anti-B

Haemolytic disease due to anti-A or anti-B is almost entirely confined to group A and B infants born to group O mothers: it is mainly group O mothers who have anti-A and anti-B of the IgG class, which can cross the placenta. ABO HDN (of all grades of severity) affects about 1 in 150 births. With the advent of successful anti-D prophylaxis, clinically significant disease is now more frequently due to anti-A or anti-B or to antibodies other than anti-D within the Rh system, or rarely to the involvement of other blood group systems. Unlike HDN due to anti-D, ABO HDN may be seen in the first pregnancy, since ABO antibodies are naturally present. ABO HDN is usually very mild; stillbirths do not occur, severe anaemia is uncommon and the child rarely requires treatment by exchange transfusion. Phototherapy is usually sufficient to reduce bilirubin levels. A consistent finding is the presence of spherocytes on inspection of cord blood smears. In certain parts of the world, ABO HDN is even more common than in the United Kingdom. This may in part result from the high concentrations of IgG anti-A and anti-B in such populations.

Blood donation and blood components

Volunteer blood donors provide red cells, platelets, plasma products and granulocytes for transfusion. This section reviews the types and uses of blood products, and the potential problems associated with transfusion.

Packed red cells are the most widely used blood product. They are given in a volume of approximately 300 ml. The great bulk of plasma is reduced, leaving approximately 20 ml; a solution of saline with

adenine, glucose and mannitol (SAG-M) is used to replace the rest of the plasma, and maintains the health of the red cells in storage. A unit of packed red cells will last for 35 days at 4°C, though stored blood tends to have reduced levels of 2,3-DPG. White cells are also routinely removed from the red cell components (leucodepleted blood).

Fresh frozen plasma (FFP) may also be prepared from whole blood donations or from apheresis collection. Blood is centrifuged to separate out the plasma and cellular phases, and the fresh plasma is frozen for up to one year. FFP is typically used to replace coagulation factor deficiencies in cases where multiple factors are lost (e.g. in disseminated intravascular coagulation with haemorrhagic symptoms, or as part of a massive transfusion protocol – see below). A slightly different product, cryoprecipitate, is rich in fibrinogen, and is prepared by thawing frozen plasma in a controlled fashion. As well as fibrinogen, other high molecular weight components are also concentrated in cryoprecipitate, including von Willebrand factor. Cryoprecipitate is an excellent product for the replacement of fibrinogen in DIC.

Platelets for transfusion may be derived from whole blood donations, again by centrifugation. A single adult dose of platelets will require the platelet component of several donors' whole blood. Platelets may also be collected by apheresis; this more efficient method allows the production of a platelet dose from a single volunteer, thus exposing the recipient to the blood of fewer individual donors. Platelets need to be stored at 22°C with constant shaking; this has been shown as the best method for maintaining their function, but increases the risk of bacterial contamination. Thus they have a relatively short shelf life of five days, and supplies need to be carefully managed.

Components more rarely used include granulocytes. The evidence for the use of granulocyte transfusions is very limited, but they are sometimes employed in severely neutropenic patients who are critically ill with sepsis, and in whom standard therapies for sepsis have failed to achieve a response. As with platelets, granulocytes may be obtained through centrifugation of whole blood or through apheresis; however, with granulocyte collections, donors must be primed with G-CSF prior to collection, to ensure that adequate numbers of cells are obtained.

Hazards of blood transfusion: The SHOT report

As with all medical interventions, the benefits of transfusion must be weighed against the associated risks. A legal framework exists to ensure the best

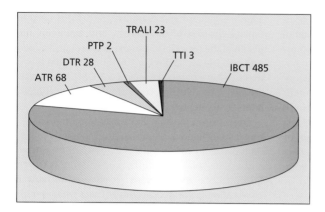

Figure 15.1 Pie chart showing hazards of transfusion in the UK from 1996–2010 as reported to the SHOT Committee. *Notes:* TRALI – transfusion-associated acute lung injury; TTI – transfusion-transmitted infection; ATR – acute transfusion reaction; DTR – delayed transfusion reaction; PTP – post-transfusion purpura; IBCT – incorrect blood component transfused

Source: UK SHOT Committee report 2010.

possible safety standards for transfusion, with regulations to monitor all aspects of collection, storage and administration. In the United Kingdom, all adverse incidents following blood transfusion are reported to the Serious Hazards of Transfusion (SHOT) Committee. The nature of the incidents and the relative frequency reported between 1996 and 2010 are given in Figure 15.1.

The commonest error reported to the SHOT Committee over this period is the transfusion of an incorrect blood product – usually a component intended for another patient. The main reasons for this are administrative – for example errors in the labelling of blood samples taken for cross-matching and the failure to match the name on the blood pack with that of the recipient. Since this raises the possibility of potentially fatal ABO-incompatible transfusions being given, strategies for reducing the risk are crucial. Some hospitals have instituted a barcoding system for blood transfusion, in which the patient's wristband and the sample taken for cross-matching are labelled with matching barcodes at the time of venepuncture. When the blood product for transfusion is chosen in the transfusion laboratory, this too is marked with the same barcode. In order for the transfusion to take place, a barcode scanner must be used to confirm that the correct product is being delivered to the correct patient – with a reduction in the likelihood of the wrong unit being administered. Simple processes such as this can significantly reduce the possibility of transfusing blood matched for another patient.

Haemolytic reactions due to incompatible red cells

The symptoms and signs that are found after a transfusion of incompatible blood depend on whether the transfused cells undergo intravascular or extravascular haemolysis. Intravascular lysis leads to haemoglobinaemia and haemoglobinuria and is almost always due to the action of anti-A or anti-B – both being strong activators of the complement system. Symptoms may appear from a few minutes to several hours after beginning to transfuse ABO-incompatible blood and may include restlessness, anxiety, fever, chills, flushing of the face, pain in the lumbar region and chest, vomiting and diarrhoea. If the reaction is severe, there is circulatory collapse and the development of acute renal failure. Sometimes, haemorrhage may occur due to disseminated intravascular coagulation.

It is not only the administration of red cells that can cause ABO incompatibility reactions. The administration of FFP or platelets with plasma that contains donor anti-A or anti-B antibodies may also lyse the recipient's own red cells if the wrong product is given to the wrong patient.

The immediate management of a mismatched transfusion is to stop the transfusion, keeping the bag and giving set so that the transfusion laboratory can check the grouping of the blood product. Circulatory support is essential and inotropes may even be needed. Sometimes furosemide may be required to try to maintain urinary output. DIC, if it develops, should be treated with standard management. When deaths do occur, they are usually the result either of severe DIC or of renal failure. The overall mortality following ABO incompatibility is probably of the order of 10%.

By contrast, when blood transfusion is followed by extravascular destruction of red cells, there are usually only chills and fever occurring one or more hours after the start of the transfusion. The most common antibody causing extravascular destruction is anti-D. This type of incompatibility is almost never followed by renal failure.

Another type of haemolytic complication is the delayed haemolytic transfusion reaction (DTR). This occurs in a recipient who has been previously immunized by transfusion or pregnancy, but in whom the plasma antibody titre has become too weak to be identified. Following the transfusion, a secondary immunological response takes place and the antibody titre rapidly rises, bringing about haemolysis, usually about seven days later. Typically, the patient develops anaemia, fever, jaundice and sometimes haemoglobinuria. Antibodies to red cell antigens Kidd (Jk) and the Rh system are the most common cause of these reactions.

Transfusion-transmitted infections

The risk of transfusion-transmitted infections (TTIs) has declined over the last decade due to the adoption of a number of safety strategies. Over the period 1996 to 2010, only 69 TTIs were reported to SHOT. The majority of TTIs are due to bacterial contamination, which is commoner in platelet components due to their storage conditions. Other theoretical TTIs include hepatitis B (HBV), human T-cell leukaemia virus (HTLV), human immunodeficiency virus (HIV) infection and hepatitis C (HCV). As would be expected, highly rigorous screening programmes are used to ensure that infected components do not enter the blood supply.

Various tiers of safety procedures have been put in place. 'Self-exclusion' is an important contributor to blood safety. Those donors who are in 'high-risk' categories are asked not to donate – for instance those who have recently travelled to a tropical country (risk of malarial transmission), and those with a history of intravenous drug abuse. Following this, testing is performed on every component donated. For hepatitis C, for example, a combination of serological tests and nucleic acid amplification tests to detect viral RNA has reduced the risk of contracting HCV from a transfusion to an estimated 1 in 22 million. A combination of serological and molecular testing is also employed to screen all samples for HBV, HIV, HTLV and syphilis, among others. The estimated chance that a blood unit infected with HIV might enter the UK supply is around 1 in 5 million, and for hepatitis B the chance is around 1 in 500 000.

A further safety procedure is the use of *pathogen inactivation technology* to inactivate viruses, bacteria, fungi and protozoa. The addition of solvent/detergent will inactivate the lipid envelope of viruses such as HBV, HCV, HIV and HTLV, and others such as Epstein–Barr virus (EBV) and cytomegalovirus (CMV). This process is only suitable for non-cellular components (e.g. intravenous immune globulin). Other methods for inactivation of pathogens include the use of photochemical systems such as psoralen-S59 compounds where, after the addition of the psoralen, the blood product is exposed to high-intensity ultraviolet A light. This technology is in use in several countries, where it has the additional advantage of prolonging the shelf life of some blood products (e.g. platelets). Bacterial infection may also be detected prior to the administration of the component through the use of technologies like Bact/Alert. This uses a gas permeable colorimetric sensor and reflected light to measure the production of CO_2 by bacterial metabolism in a blood component product. As CO_2 levels climb, the colour of the BactAlert vial turns yellow, increasing reflectance, and allowing detection of the earliest stages of bacterial infection. Frequent monitoring using this system will limit the number of potentially infected units that enter the supply.

Variant Creutzfeldt–Jakob disease

CJD is one of a group of transmissible spongiform encephalopathy disorders, and it exists in familial, sporadic and variant types. The pathogenic agent is believed to be a prion protein, which causes disease by affecting the normal conformation of other proteins. There is a long incubation period and so far there is no treatment for the progressive, central nervous system degeneration that this condition produces. Rapidly progressive dementia is followed by early death. Particular concern arose regarding the variant form of CJD during the outbreak of bovine spongiform encephalopathy (BSE) in cattle in the United Kingdom in the 1980s. This sparked considerable concern about the possibility of transmission of the responsible prion through the food chain, with the development of the disease after consuming beef from affected cattle. The long incubation period raised the spectre of many potentially infected yet asymptomatic people.

It was also reported that v-CJD can be transmitted by blood transfusion. As a precaution, UK blood services exclude any potential blood donors who received blood products from or gave blood to individuals who subsequently developed v-CJD, or who have received a blood transfusion since 1980. In addition, all units of blood are leuco depleted to reduce potentially infected white cells from donors transmitting the disease. There is currently no screening test for v-CJD.

Cytomegalovirus

CMV is a DNA herpes virus associated with leucocytes, and may be transmitted via respiratory secretions, sexually and during childbirth. The incidence of CMV antibodies varies in different parts of the world, from 30% to 80% or more. As with most herpes viruses, the virus persists latently after infection.

In immunocompetent people, the disease caused by CMV varies from a subclinical infection to the appearance of lymphadenopathy and a mild hepatitis. The main danger of CMV infection is in infants and immunocompromised patients and thus prevention of CMV infection through blood transfusion is targeted to defined patient groups. Premature neonates of low birth weight born to mothers without anti-CMV antibody are especially at risk. Patients receiving bone marrow and solid organ transplants are also at risk (see Chapter 12). Thus CMV-antibody negative blood is generally made available for these patients, although leucodepletion (which is now standard) may offer a similar degree of protection against transfusion-transmitted CMV infection.

Other infections

Other infections known to be transmitted by transfusion include syphilis and malaria. The prevention of transmission of syphilis is by serological testing of donors. Another factor of importance is the storage of blood at 4°C, since spirochaetes do not survive for more than a few days under these conditions. With regard to malaria, individuals who have returned from an area where malaria is endemic are not accepted as donors for six months. Anyone with a positive malaria antibody test (MAT) is routinely debarred from donation. Brucellosis, babesiosis, Chagas' disease (caused by *Trypanosoma cruzi*), West Nile virus (prevalent in the USA and Canada) and parvovirus B19, which is not inactivated by detergent methods, have also been transmitted by transfusion.

As new diseases emerge from time to time, the risk of TTI always remains. It is therefore important that transfusion is only given when essential for survival or quality of life, so that the benefits clearly outweigh the uncertain risks of TTI.

Transfusion-associated graft versus host disease

Transfusion of viable white cells in blood products can in very rare circumstances lead to transfusion-associated graft versus host disease (TA-GVHD). This typically fatal disorder is seen in patients with compromised immune function, but may also occur when a patient receives a blood component from a donor who shares an HLA haplotype. Either of these situations mean that the transfused lymphocytes are not cleared in the normal way, but can engraft and function in the recipient, leading to a clinical picture that usually includes a rash and marrow failure. It can be eliminated by irradiating the blood products (red cells, platelets or plasma) before administration. Patients undergoing bone marrow transplantation, those with Hodgkin lymphoma and patients who have received purine analogue chemotherapy (e.g. fludarabine) are among those who should receive only irradiated blood products to avoid this complication.

Immediate-type hypersensitivity

Hypersensitivity reactions may occur soon after the transfusion of blood or plasma. The antibodies involved are often unknown, but some severe reactions are caused by anti-IgA antibodies. IgA deficiency is uncommon, but patients who lack IgA, and who have previously been sensitized to this immunoglobulin, may manifest allergic reactions if IgA-containing blood products are administered. In mild cases, features may be limited to urticaria, erythema, maculopapular rash or periorbital oedema. In the more severe reactions, hypotension may occur; bronchospasm and laryngeal oedema are rare.

Mild hypersensitivity reactions of any cause probably occur in about 1–3% of transfusions and can be treated with antihistamines. Severe reactions are very infrequent (1:20 000) and these may require the administration of hydrocortisone and adrenaline.

Transfusion-related acute lung injury (TRALI)

This complication typically arises after the transfusion of plasma-rich blood components, and is thought to be due to the interaction of donor anti-leucocyte antibodies in the transfused blood component interacting with the recipient's leucocytes. However, a comprehensive understanding of the pathogenesis of TRALI has not yet been established. Additional 'hits' are thought to be needed in order for the clinical picture to emerge, since TRALI is most often seen in patients already ill with pulmonary pathology.

The symptoms and signs of TRALI typically arise within six hours of transfusion, with dyspnoea and hypotension being accompanied by bilateral infiltrates on the chest x-ray. The differential diagnosis of pulmonary oedema is best excluded by examining the central venous pressure: while in fluid overload it is high, in TRALI it would be expected to be low. Management is supportive, and donors from whom implicated blood products were prepared are excluded from donating further components.

Circulatory overload

Circulatory overload with consequent cardiac failure can easily be brought about by the too-rapid transfusion of blood, especially in the elderly and in those who have been severely anaemic for some time. The first signs are dyspnoea, crepitations at the lung bases and a rise in jugular venous pressure. Stopping the transfusion is the first therapeutic manoeuvre, followed by diuresis if needed. The rate at which blood is transfused must be tailored to the urgency of the clinical situation and the cardiovascular fitness of the patient.

Citrate toxicity

Citrate toxicity is due to the reduction in ionized calcium in the patient's plasma, and may cause significant problems if large volumes of stored blood need to be given rapidly. The typical signs are tremors and prolongation of the QT interval in the electrocardiogram. Very high rates of transfusion may warrant consideration of calcium gluconate administration to avoid this complication.

Other hazards

Prior to the universal leucodepletion of blood products, febrile reactions occurred in 0.5–1% of transfusions. Reactions were due to the presence of pyrogens (e.g. soluble bacterial polysaccharides) in the anticoagulant, or to the presence in the recipient of anti-HLA antibodies or granulocyte-specific antibodies, resulting from immunization during pregnancy or previous transfusions. Both are now uncommon.

Management of transfusion reactions

The first diagnosis to exclude is an acute haemolytic transfusion reaction. Thus, in any patient with fever, tachycardia hypotension, dyspnoea or chest/abdominal pain, the first action is always to stop the transfusion and clarify that the correct patient's details are on the component being transfused. Any suspicion of ABO incompatibility should

lead to the institution of circulatory support with IV fluids, careful monitoring of pulse, blood pressure and urine output, and supportive management of any developing DIC. The component bag should be returned to the transfusion laboratory with a fresh cross-match sample from the patient; if incompatible cells have been transfused, they may still be detectable in the patient's blood. Samples should also be sent to assess for intravascular haemolysis – including a full blood count, serum haptoglobin, and haemoglobinuria.

Other haemolytic reactions, although unlikely to be as severe, should be managed in similar fashion. It is important to ensure that the possibility of bacterially contaminated units has been addressed through taking blood cultures. If necessary, broad-spectrum antibiotics may be commenced empirically after cultures have been drawn.

Severe allergic reaction should be treated initially by stopping the transfusion and returning the unit to the laboratory, as above. Chlorpheniramine may help, but severe reactions are likely to require oxygen and nebulized salbutamol, plus intramuscular adrenaline in the case of circulatory collapse.

In addition to the reactions described above, acute dyspnoea can occur due to circulatory overload (with an elevated venous pressure being a key physical sign) and in TRALI. Diuresis is clearly indicated in the former, while the latter is treated supportively, with ventilatory support where needed.

With mild fevers only, simple interventions may suffice (e.g. giving an antipyretic and slowing the transfusion); similarly, if a mild allergic reaction is evident (e.g. urticaria), chlorpheniramine followed by a slower reinstatement of the transfusion may help.

Delayed transfusion reactions may be harder to diagnose and investigate, since the temporal association with the transfusion is lost. However, it is still important to establish the nature of the reaction so that future transfusions may be managed effectively. Appropriate investigations include a full blood count, a direct antiglobulin test, serum bilirubin and assessment of renal function. Treatment is rarely needed, but the expected rise in haemoglobin after transfusion may not be seen.

Massive transfusion

Patients with acute haemorrhage (i.e. loss of red cells and plasma) may need to be transfused with large quantities of packed red cells. Massive transfusion has been defined as the replacement of one blood volume over 24 hours, or as the replacement of 50% of circulating volume in 3 hours. In such emergencies, it is critical that there is good communication between the clinicians responsible for the patient and the staff of the blood transfusion laboratory. Group compatible blood can usually be available within 15 minutes of a cross-match sample arriving in the laboratory, obviating the need for 'universal donor' group O RhD-negative blood. With the transfusion of many units of packed red cells, the patient may become deficient in key plasma components such as clotting factors and may also become thrombocytopenic (even in the absence of DIC). There is limited evidence to guide transfusion practice in this field, but the administration of one unit of FFP per unit of red cells may be effective in replacing clotting factors. Fibrinogen and platelets should also be replaced, with 2 pools of cryoprecipitate and 1 adult dose of platelets per 6–8 units of packed red cells. Wherever possible, this general approach should be personalized by laboratory testing of the full blood count and coagulation profile.

16

Further reading

General reference books

Bain, B.J. (2006) *Blood Cells: A Practical Guide.* Oxford: Wiley-Blackwell.

Bain, B.J., Bates, I., Laffan, M.A. & Lewis, S.M. (2012) *Dacie and Lewis Practical Haematology*, 11th edn. Amsterdam: Elsevier.

Hoffbrand, V., Pettit, J.E. & Vyas, P. (2009) *Color Atlas of Clinical Hematology*, 4th edn. Amsterdam: Elsevier Health.

Kaushansky, K., Lichtman, M.A., Beutler, E., Kipps, T.J., Prchal, J. & Seligsohn, U. (2010) *Williams Hematology*, 8th edn. New York: McGraw-Hill.

Orkin, S.H., Nathan, D.G., Ginsburg, D., Look, A.T., Fisher, D.E. & Lux IV, S. (2008) *Nathan and Oski's Hematology of Infancy and Childhood: Expert Consult: Online and Print*, 7th edn. Philadelphia: Saunders Publishing.

Swerdlow, S.H., Campo, E., Harris, N.L., Jaffe, E.S., Pileri, S.A., Stein, H., Thiele, J. & Vardiman, J.W. (2008) *WHO Classification of Tumours of Haematopoietic and Lymphoid Tissue*, 4th edn. Geneva: WHO Press.

Chapter 1 An introduction to haematopoiesis

Kaushansky, K.N. (2006) Mechanisms of disease: Lineage-specific hematopoietic growth factors, *New England Journal of Medicine*, May 11; 354: 2034–2045.

Orkin, S.H. & Zon, L.I. (2008) Hematopoiesis: An evolving paradigm for stem cell biology, *Cell*, February 22; 132(4): 631–644.

Osawa, M., Hanada, J., Hamada, H., & Nakauchi, H. (1996) Long-term lymphohematopoietic reconstitution by a single CD34-low/negative hematopoietic stem cell, *Science*, July 12; 273(5272): 242–245.

Palis, J. (2008) Ontogeny of erythropoiesis, *Current Opinion in Hematology*, May; 15(3): 155–161.

Zhu, J. & Emerson, G. (2002) Hematopoietic cytokines, transcription factors and lineage commitment, *Oncogene*, 21(21): 3295–3313.

Chapter 2 Anaemia: General principles

Fleming, R.E. & Ponka, P.N. (2012) Iron overload in human disease, *New England Journal of Medicine*, January 26; 366(4): 348–359.

Ganz, T. & Nemeth, E. (2011) The hepcidin-ferroportin system as a therapeutic target in anemias and iron overload disorders, *Hematology: American Society of Hematology Education Program*, 2011: 538–542.

Goonewardene, M., Shehata, M. & Hamad, A. (2012) Best Practice and Research: *Clinical Obstetrics and Gynaecology*, February; 26(1): 3–24.

Kaferle, J. & Strzoda, C.E. (2009) Evaluation of macrocytosis, *American Family Physician*, Feb 1; 79(3): 203–208.

Lankhorst, C.E. & Wish, J.B. (2010) Anemia in renal disease: Diagnosis and management, *Blood Reviews*, Jan; 24(1): 39–47.

Liu, K. & Kaffes, A.J. (2012) Iron deficiency anaemia: A review of diagnosis, investigation and management, *European Journal of Gastroenterology and Hepatology*, February; 24(2): 109–116.

Roy, C.N. (2010) Anemia of inflammation, *Hematology: American Society for Hematology Education Program*, 2010: 276–280.

Solomon, L.R. (2007) Disorders of cobalamin (vitamin B12) metabolism: Emerging concepts in pathophysiology, diagnosis and treatment, *Blood Reviews*, May; 21(3): 113–130.

Weiss, G. & Goodnough, L.T. (2005) Medical progress: Anemia of chronic disease, *New England Journal of Medicine*, 352: 1011–1023.

Haematology Lecture Notes, Ninth edition. C.S.R. Hatton, N.C. Hughes-Jones, D. Hay and D. Keeling. © 2013 John Wiley & Sons, Ltd. Published 2013 by John Wiley & Sons, Ltd.

Chapter 3 Haemolytic anaemias

An, X. & Mohandas, N. (2008) Disorders of red cell membrane. British Journal of Haematology, May; 141(3): 367–375.

Barcellini, W., Bianchi, P., Fermo, E., Imperiali, F.G., Marcello, A.P., Vercellati, C., Zaninoni, A. & Zanella, A. (2011) Hereditary red cell membrane defects: Diagnostic and clinical aspects, *Blood Transfusion*, July; 9(3): 274–277.

Bruce, L.J. (2008) *Red cell membrane transport abnormalities, Current Opinion in Hematology*, May; 15(3): 184–190.

Fibach, E. & Rachmilewitz, E. (2008) The role of oxidative stress in hemolytic anemia, *Current Molecular Medicine*, Nov; 8(7): 609–619.

Garratty, G. (2009) Drug-induced immune hemolytic anemia, *Hematology: American Society for Hematology Education Program*, 2009: 73–79.

Hoffman, P.C. (2009) Immune hemolytic anemia: Selected topics, *Hematology: American Society for Hematology Education Program*, 2009: 80–86.

Parker, C.J. (2008) Paroxysmal nocturnal hemoglobinuria: An historical overview, *Hematology: American Society for Hematology Education Program*, 2008: 93–103.

Petz, L.D. (2008) Cold antibody autoimmune hemolytic anemias, *Blood Review*, Jan; 22(1): 1–15.

Tavazzi, D., Taher, A. & Cappellini, M.D. (2008) Red blood cell enzyme disorders: An overview, *Pediatric Annals*, May; 37(5): 303–310.

Chapter 4 Disorders of globin synthesis

Bauer, D.E. & Orkin, S.H. (2011) Update on fetal hemoglobin gene regulation in hemoglobinopathies, *Current Opinion in Pediatrics*, Feb; 23(1): 1–8.

Bunn, H.F., Nathan, D.G., Dover, G.J., Hebbel, R.P., Platt, O.S., Rosse, W.F. & Ware, R.E. (2010) Pulmonary hypertension and nitric oxide depletion in sickle cell disease, *Blood*, August 5; 116(5): 687–692.

Higgs, D.R., Engel, J.D. & Stamatoyannopoulos, G. (2012) Thalassaemia, *Lancet,* January 28; 379(9813): 373–383.

Paul, R.N., Castro, O.L., Aggarwal, A. & Oneal, P.A. (2011) Acute chest syndrome: Sickle cell disease, *European Journal of Haematology*, September; 87(3): 191–207.

Rees, D.C., Williams, T.N. & Gladwin, M.T. (2010) Sickle-cell disease, *Lancet*, December 11; 376(9757): 2018–2031.

Verduzco, L.A. & Nathan, D.G. (2009) Sickle cell disease and stroke, *Blood*, December 10; 114(25): 5117–5125.

Chapters 5 to 13 Malignant haematology, aplastic anaemia and pure red cell aplasia

Swerdlow et al. (2008), detailed in General reference books above, provides a very clear, concise reference for all the haematological malignancies and related disorders, and is highly recommended to those students of haematology who require greater detail, particularly with regard to the pathology and genetics of the disorders. For students requiring more information with regard to management and treatment, the following references are recommended.

Campbell, P.J., Maclean, C., Beer, P.A., Buck, G., Wheatley, K., Kiladjian, J.J. et al. (2012) Correlation of blood counts with vascular complications in essential thrombocythemia: Analysis of the prospective PT1 cohort, *Blood*, August 16; 120(7): 1409–1411.

Cavalli, F., Isaacson, P.G., Gascoyne, R.D. & Zucca, E. (2001) MALT lymphomas, *Hematology: American Society of Hematology Education Program*, 2001: 241–258.

Cervantes, F., Dupriez, B., Passamonti, F., Vannucchi, A.M., Morra, E., Reilly, J.T. et al. (2012) Improving survival trends in primary myelofibrosis: An international study, *Journal of Clinical Oncology*, August 20, 30: 2981–2987.

Chakraverty, R. & Mackinnion, S. (2011) Allogeneic transplantation for lymphoma, *Journal of Clinical Oncology*, May 10; 29(14): 1855–1863.

Coiffier, B., Lepage, E., Briere, J., Herbrecht, R., Tilly, H., Bouabdallah, R. et al. (2002) CHOP chemotherapy plus rituximab compared with CHOP alone in elderly patients with diffuse large-B-cell lymphoma, *New England Journal of Medicine*, 346(4): 235–242.

Craddock, C. (2000) Haemopoietic stem-cell transplantation: Recent progress and future promise, *Lancet Oncology*, December; 1: 227–234.

Deng, C., Lee, S. & O'Connor, O.A. (2012) New strategies in the treatment of mantle cell lymphoma, *Clinical Cancer Research*, 18(13): 3499–3508.

Eich, H.T., Diehl, V., Görgen, H., Pabst, T., Markova, J., Debus, J. et al. (2010) Intensified chemotherapy and dose-reduced involved-field radiotherapy in patients with early unfavorable Hodgkin's lymphoma: Final analysis of the German Hodgkin Study Group HD11 trial, *Journal of Clinical Oncology*, 28: 4199–4206.

Evens, A.M., Hutchings, M. & Diehl, V. (2008) Treatment of Hodgkin lymphoma: The past, present, and future, *National Clinical Practice Oncology*, 5: 543–556.

Fields, P.A. & Linch, D.C. (2012) Treatment of the elderly patient with diffuse large B-cell lymphoma, *British Journal of Haematology*, 157: 159–170.

Harrison, C.N. & Green, A.R. (2006) Essential thrombocythaemia, *Best Practice and Research: Clinical Haematology*, 19: 439–453.

Jaffe, E.S. & Pittaluga, S. (2011) Aggressive B-cell lymphomas: A review of new and old entities in the WHO classification, *Hematology: American Society for Hematology Education Program*, 2011: 506–514.

Li, L., Bierman, P., Vose, J., Loberiza, F., Armitage, J.O. & Bociek, R.G. (2011) High-dose therapy/autologous hematopoietic stem cell transplantation in relapsed or refractory marginal zone non-Hodgkin lymphoma, *Clinical Lymphoma, Myeloma and Leukemia*, 11: 253–256.

Linch, D.C. (2011) Burkitt lymphoma in adults, *British Journal of Haematology*, 156: 693–703.

Mahindra, A., Laubach, L., Raje, N., Munshi, N., Richardson, P.G. & Anderson, K. (2012) Latest advances and current challenges in the treatment of multiple myeloma, *Nature Reviews: Clinical Oncology*, 9: 135–143.

Marcus, R., Imrie, K., Solal-Celigny, P., Catalano, J.V., Dmoszunska, A., Raposo, J.C. et al. (2008) Phase III study of R-CVP compared with cyclophosphamide, vincristine, and prednisone alone in patients with previously untreated advanced follicular lymphoma, *Journal of Clinical Oncology*, 26: 4579–4586.

Michallet, A.-S., Coiffier, B. & Salles, G. (2011) Maintenance therapy in follicular lymphoma, *Current Opinion in Oncology*, 23(5): 449–454.

Moreau, P., Richardson, P.G., Cavo, M., Orlowski, R.Z., San Miguel, J.F., Palumbo, A. & Harousseau, J.L. (2012) Proteasome inhibitors in multiple myeloma: 10 years later, *Blood*, 120: 947–959.

Moskowitz, C. (2012) Diffuse large B Cell lymphoma: How can we cure more patients in 2012? *Best Practice and Research in Clinical Haematology*, 25(1): 41–47.

Passamonti, F. (2012) How I treat polycythemia vera, *Blood*, 120: 275–284.

Tang, T., Tay, K., Quek, R., Tao, M., Tan, S.Y., Tan, L., & Lim, S.T. (2010) Peripheral T-cell lymphoma: Review and updates of current management strategies, *Advances in Hematology*, 2010: 1–8.

Tefferi, A. (2011) Primary myelofibrosis: 2012 update on diagnosis, risk stratification, and management, *American Journal of Hematology*, 86: 1017–1026.

Weisenburger, D.D., Savage, K.J., Harris, N.L., Gascoyne, R.D., Jaffe, E.S., MacLennan, K.A. et al. (2011) Peripheral T-cell lymphoma, not otherwise specified: A report of 340 cases from the International Peripheral T-cell Lymphoma Project, *Blood*, 117(12): 3402–3408.

Wündisch, T., Thiede, C., Morgner, A., Dempfle, A., Günther, A., Liu, H. et al. (2005) Long-term follow-up of gastric MALT lymphoma after Helicobacter pylori eradication, *Journal of Clinical Oncology*, 23(31): 8018–8024.

Chapter 14 Haemostasis, abnormal bleeding and anticoagulant therapy

Baglin, T., Gray, E., Greaves, M., Hunt, B.J., Keeling, D., Machin, S. et al. (2010) Clinical guidelines for testing for heritable thrombophilia, *British Journal of Haematology*, 149: 209–220.

Cuker, A. & Cines, D.B. (2012) How I treat heparin-induced thrombocytopenia, *Blood*, 119: 2209–2218.

George, J.N. (2010) How I treat patients with thrombotic thrombocytopenic purpura: 2010, *Blood*, 116: 4060–4069.

Guyatt, G.H., Akl, E.A., Crowther, M., Schunemann, H.J., Gutterman, D.D., Zelman Lewis, S. & American College of Chest, P. (2012) Introduction to the ninth edition: Antithrombotic Therapy and Prevention of Thrombosis, 9th ed: American College of Chest Physicians Evidence-Based Clinical Practice Guidelines, *Chest*, 141: 48S–52S.

Hay, C.R., Brown, S., Collins, P.W., Keeling, D.M. & Liesner, R. (2006) The diagnosis and management of factor VIII and IX inhibitors: A guideline from the United Kingdom Haemophilia Centre Doctors Organisation, *British Journal of Haematology*, 133: 591–605.

Keeling, D., Baglin, T., Tait, C., Watson, H., Perry, D., Baglin, C., Kitchen, S. & Makris, M. (2011) Guidelines on oral anticoagulation with warfarin, fourth edition, *British Journal of Haematology*, 154: 311–324.

Keeling, D., Mackie, I., Moore, G.W., Greer, I.A., Greaves, M. & British Committee for Standards in, H. (2012) Guidelines on the investigation and management of antiphospholipid syndrome, *British Journal of Haematology*, Feb 8, doi: 10.1111/j.1365-2141.2012.09037.x.

Levi, M., Toh, C.H., Thachil, J. & Watson, H.G. (2009) Guidelines for the diagnosis and management of disseminated intravascular coagulation. British Committee for Standards in Haematology, *British Journal of Haematology*, 145: 24–33.

Provan, D., Stasi, R., Newland, A.C., Blanchette, V.S., Bolton-Maggs, P., Bussel, J.B. et al. (2010) International consensus report on the investigation and management of primary immune thrombocytopenia, *Blood*, 115: 168–186.

Rodeghiero, F., Castaman, G. & Tosetto, A. (2009) How I treat von Willebrand disease, *Blood*, 114: 1158–1165.

Chapter 15 Blood groups and blood transfusion

Alter, H.J. & Klein, H.G. (2008) The hazards of blood transfusion in historical perspective, *Blood*, October 1; 112(7): 2617–2626.

Anstee, D.J. (2009) Red cell genotyping and the future of pretransfusion testing, *Blood*, July 9; 114(2): 248–256.

Brinc, D. & Lazarus, A.H. (2009) Mechanisms of anti-D action in the prevention of hemolytic disease of the fetus and newborn, *Hematology: American Society for Hematology Education Program*, 2009: 185–191.

Egbor, M., Knott, P. & Bhide, A. (2012) Red-cell and platelet alloimmunisation in pregnancy, *Best Practice and Research in Clinical Obstetric Gynaecology*, Febuary; 26(1): 119–132.

Isbister, J.P., Shander, A., Spahn, D.R., Erhard, J., Farmer, S.L. & Hofmann, A. (2011) Adverse blood transfusion outcomes: Establishing causation, *Transfusion Medicine Reviews*, April; 25(2): 89–101.

Kim, Y.A. & Makar, R.S. (2012) *Detection of fetomaternal hemorrhage*, American Journal of Hematology, April; 87(4): 417–423.

Klein, H.G. & Anstee, D.J. (2007) *Mollison's Blood Tranfusion in Clinical Medicine*, 11th edn, Oxford: Wiley-Blackwell.

McClelland, D.B.L. (2007) *Handbook of Transfusion Medicine*, 4th edn, Norwich: United Kingdom Blood Services, available at http://www.transfusionguidelines.org.uk/index.aspx?publication=htm, accessed 11 September 2011.

Sachs, U.J. (2011) Recent insights into the mechanism of transfusion-related acute lung injury, *Current Opinion in Hematology*, November; 18(6): 436–442.

SHOT, http://www.shotuk.org/home/, the Serious Hazards of Transfusion Scheme of the NHS blood and transplant service, accessed 11 September 2011.

Index

Haematology Lecture Notes, Ninth edition. C.S.R. Hatton, N.C. Hughes-Jones, D. Hay and D. Keeling. © 2013 John Wiley & Sons, Ltd.
Published 2013 by John Wiley & Sons, Ltd.